The Canker Sore Mastery Bible: Your Blueprint for Complete Canker Sore Management

Dr. Ankita Kashyap and Prof. Krishna N. Sharma

Published by Virtued Press, 2023.

While every precaution has been taken in the preparation of this book, the publisher assumes no responsibility for errors or omissions, or for damages resulting from the use of the information contained herein.

THE CANKER SORE MASTERY BIBLE: YOUR BLUEPRINT FOR COMPLETE CANKER SORE MANAGEMENT

First edition. December 20, 2023.

Copyright © 2023 Dr. Ankita Kashyap and Prof. Krishna N. Sharma.

ISBN: 979-8223558538

Written by Dr. Ankita Kashyap and Prof. Krishna N. Sharma.

Table of Contents

....	1
Introduction	2
Understanding Canker Sores	5
Defining Canker Sores	6
Symptoms and Signs	11
Canker Sores Vs. Cold Sores	20
The Impact on Daily Life	24
Myth-Busting: Common Misconceptions	27
When to Seek Medical Attention	30
The Science Behind Canker Sores	33
Genetic Factors and Predisposition	34
Nutritional Deficiencies Linked to Canker Sores	36
The Role of Stress and Hormones	39
Immunological Aspects	42
Epidemiology: Who Gets Canker Sores?	45
Current Research and Developments	48
Medical Treatments for Canker Sores	51
Topical Medications: Types and Usage	52
Oral Medications: A Deeper Dive	57
Corticosteroid Treatments: Pros and Cons	62
Pain Management Strategies	67
The Role of Antibiotics in Treatment	70
When to Consider Cauterization	73
Immunosuppressants and Canker Sores	76
Diagnosis and Professional Care	79
Working With Your Dentist or Doctor	80
Understanding Medications and Prescriptions	82
When Surgery Is Considered	85
The Role of Dental Hygiene	88
Insurance and Cost Considerations	90
Diet and Nutrition: The Canker Sore Connection	93

Foods to Avoid: Canker Sore Culprits..94
Healing Foods: What to Eat When You Have a Canker Sore. 99
Vitamins and Supplements for Prevention 102
The Role of Hydration in Canker Sore Management...............105
Understanding Food Allergies and Sensitivities 108
Anti-inflammatory Diets and Canker Sores 111
Meal Planning for Canker Sore Management 114
Holistic and Alternative Approaches 117
Herbal Remedies 118
Acupuncture and Acupressure...123
Aromatherapy and Essential Oils..128
Homeopathy and Canker Sores 133
Stress Management Techniques..138
Nutritional Supplements..142
The Mind-Body Connection 145
Lifestyle Modifications for Canker Sore Prevention 148
The Importance of Oral Hygiene 149
Sleep and Canker Sores: The Restorative Connection 152
Exercise: Boosting Immunity and Reducing Outbreaks 155
Avoiding Oral Trauma..158
Quitting Smoking: A Path to Better Oral Health.................161
Managing Hormonal Fluctuations 164
Environmental Factors and Canker Sores 167
Psychological Approaches to Canker Sore Management......170
Mindfulness and Meditation for Stress Reduction 171
Biofeedback: Controlling the Pain Response........................174
The Impact of Positive Affirmations.....................................176
Art Therapy: A Creative Outlet for Healing 181
Journaling for Emotional Release and Tracking...................184
Self-Care and Home Remedies 188
Over-the-Counter Solutions 189
Rinses and Washes...193
Topical Applications 196

Managing Pain and Discomfort 200
Healing Boosters...205
Preventive Measures at Home..210
When Home Remedies Aren't Enough 215
Customizing Your Canker Sore Management Plan 221
Assessing Your Individual Triggers..222
Creating a Tailored Diet Plan 225
Selecting the Right Supplements...229
Integrating Holistic Practices Into Daily Life.............................233
Designing a Stress Management Program 236
Monitoring and Adapting Your Plan..239
When to Seek Professional Help..242
Navigating Social Situations...245
Dining Out With Dietary Restrictions 246
Explaining Canker Sores to Others 249
Social Eating Strategies..252
Networking and Professional Settings 255
Romantic Relationships and Intimacy...257
Traveling With Canker Sores..259
Canker Sores and Public Speaking..262
Pediatric Canker Sores: A Parent's Guide 265
Recognizing Canker Sores in Children 266
Treatment Options for Children 269
Communicating With Your Child's Healthcare Provider 272
Soothing Techniques for Children 275
Nutritional Considerations for Kids 277
Supporting Your Child's Emotional Health 280
Educating Peers and Caregivers...283
Advanced Topics in Canker Sore Research................................286
Emerging Therapies..287
Genetic Studies and Personalized Medicine...............................290
The Microbiome and Canker Sores 293
Immunotherapy and Canker Sores...297

Regenerative Medicine and Healing 301
International Approaches to Canker Sores 305
Future Directions in Canker Sore Management 309

DISCLAIMER

The information provided in this book is intended for general informational purposes only. The content is not meant to substitute professional medical advice, diagnosis, or treatment. Always consult with a qualified healthcare provider before making any changes to your management plan or healthcare regimen.

While every effort has been made to ensure the accuracy and completeness of the information presented, the author and publisher do not assume any responsibility for errors, omissions, or potential misinterpretations of the content. Individual responses to management strategies may vary, and what works for one person might not be suitable for another.

The book does not endorse any specific medical treatments, products, or services. Readers are encouraged to seek guidance from their healthcare providers to determine the most appropriate approaches for their unique medical conditions and needs.

Any external links or resources provided in the book are for convenience and informational purposes only. The author and publisher do not have control over the content or availability of these external sources and do not endorse or guarantee the accuracy of such information.

Readers are advised to exercise caution and use their judgment when applying the information provided in this book to their own situations. The author and publisher disclaim any liability for any direct, indirect, consequential, or other damages arising from the use of this book and its content.

Introduction

Setting off on an adventure through the maze-like realm of health and healing, especially when it comes to a condition as nettlesome as canker sores, can be unsettling and uncomfortable. Millions of people walk this journey, but it is frequently done so in quiet and under the shadow of more well-known health problems. However, the fight to conquer this ailment is urgent for people who experience the constant sting and sharp of these little but powerful oral lesions.

This book began in a quiet nook of a library, surrounded by tall volumes of medical journals and texts. These pages are the result of a painstaking compilation of research, facts, and firsthand accounts. The Canker Sore Mastery Bible is a beacon that shines through the mist of doubt and shows the path to a life free from the burden of canker sores, not just another collection of repeated facts.

How many times have you experienced the first tingle and realised, with a tired acceptance, that the next few days would be characterised by the discomfort and annoyance of a fresh sore? How many times have you searched the internet for a cure-all only to be confronted with a deluge of unsubstantiated claims and contradicting guidance? There is none of that kind of uncertainty in this book. Rather, you will find a comprehensive management guide for canker sores that has been painstakingly designed to meet your needs and provide you with information.

This strategy is comprehensive but firmly based in science. The biological causes of canker sores as well as potential environmental and psychological triggers are revealed in each chapter, which opens up like the petals of a healing flower. This book aims to provide you, the reader, with a thorough understanding of the disease so that you may make educated decisions regarding your health rather than just listing cures.

When was the last time you enjoyed a meal without having to worry about experiencing pain? Have you ever wished that day might come back to you as a new normal rather than just a passing thought? The methods outlined here are designed to be practical, giving you not only the "what," but also the "how" of managing canker sores. They are instruments, refined by the experiences of those who have gone before you and fortified by years of intense study.

In keeping with the accessibility theme, the language used is deliberate and free of the complex medical jargon that frequently turns off the people it is meant to assist. Rather, simplicity and clarity serve as the compass, preventing complexity from entangling the wisdom that is present. Every sentence is carefully constructed to move you closer to mastery and every word is picked with purpose.

Personalization is essential. Since it is crucial to acknowledge individuality, the management plans that are offered are not all-inclusive. They are adaptable and made to fit the particular fabric of your life. This book respects the fact that every person is unique and provides a range of answers, from naturally holistic to traditional medical approaches.

Do you think it's possible to live a life free of canker sores? When the grin in the mirror is free of the obvious symptoms of this illness, is it possible for you to picture that day? Not only is there hope, but there is also a concrete plan and a set of actions that, if followed, can result in that exact result.

I want you to actively interact with the content as you turn each page. Pose inquiries to the text and, consequently, to yourself. Let your scepticism help you and your curiosity lead the way. There is a place where mastery seeds are sown and understanding grows in the conversation between the writer and the reader.

This book is your guide, your friend, and maybe even your comfort. It is a single, unrelenting purpose and the result of innumerable hours of research—to give you the tools you need to take charge of your canker sores and recover the quality of life you deserve.

    Let us begin.

Understanding Canker Sores

Defining Canker Sores

Traveling through the maze-like realm of health and recovery, especially when it comes to a condition as nettlesome as canker sores, can be an uncomfortable and difficult journey. Millions walk this journey, but it's frequently in quiet alone, hidden by the shadow of more serious health problems. But for individuals who live with the constant pain and sting of these tiny but powerful mouth lesions, beating back this ailment is a vital battle.

The origins of this book were found in the peaceful nook of a library, amidst the tall volumes of medical journals and texts. The pages that are in front of you are a carefully curated collection of facts, research, and first-hand accounts. The Canker Sore Mastery Bible is not just another collection of recycled material; rather, it is a lighthouse that shines through the mist of doubt and shows the path to a life free from the burden of canker sores.

How often has the first twinge occurred and you knew, with a tired resignation, that the next few days will bring the annoyance and agony of a fresh sore? When searching for a cure online, how often have you been confronted with a deluge of unsubstantiated claims and contradicting guidance? You won't encounter any such ambiguity in this book. Rather, you will find a recipe for managing canker sores in their entirety—a manual that has been painstakingly designed to meet your needs and provide you with information.

Here, a comprehensive yet firmly scientific approach is adopted. The chapters expand in a manner like to a healing flower's petals, exposing not only the biological foundations of canker sores but also the potential influences of environmental and psychological variables. Instead than just listing treatments, the goal of this book is to provide you, the reader, with a thorough understanding of the illness so that you can make educated decisions regarding your own health.

When was the last time you enjoyed a meal without the fear of suffering hanging over you? Have you ever wished that day might come back to you, not as a passing memory but as a brand-new standard? You will learn not just the "what," but also the "how" of managing canker sores from the actionable techniques outlined here. They are instruments that have been refined by the experiences of those who have gone before you and forged in the furnace of intense investigation.

The language used is deliberate and free of the complex medical jargon that frequently turns off the people it is intended to assist, all in the spirit of accessibility. Rather, simplicity and clarity serve as the guiding principles, making sure that complication does not entangle the wisdom that is contained within. Every word has been picked carefully, and every sentence is designed to move you closer to mastery.

Tailoring is essential. Since individuality is highly valued, the management plans that are offered are not all-inclusive. They can be shaped to fit the particular fabric of your life since they are flexible. A range of answers, from the medically conventional to the organically holistic, is provided in this book to acknowledge the fact that what works for one person may not work for another.

Are you of the opinion that living a life free of canker sores is possible? Is there a day you can picture a grin in the mirror that is free of the obvious symptoms of this illness? Herein lies not only hope but also a concrete plan of action, a set of procedures that, when followed, can bring about that very result.

As you go through the pages, I encourage you to actively interact with the information. Inquire not only of the text but also of yourself in general. Give in to your scepticism and let your curiosity lead the way. There is an interaction between the writer and the reader where mastery seeds are sown and understanding grows.

This book serves as a friend, a guide, and possibly a comfort. It is the result of innumerable hours of research and the embodiment of one steadfast commitment: to provide you the tools you need to take charge of your canker sores and recover the quality of life you deserve.

Before we delve into the , it is essential to provide a clear and organized listing of the words that are fundamental to understanding canker sores. By setting clear expectations for the reader, we aim to foster an environment of informed exploration and learning. The following terms will be explored in detail:

1. Canker Sores
2. Aphthous Stomatitis
3. Etiology
4. Triggers
5. Immune Response
6. Ulceration
7. Oral Mucosa
8. Recurrence

1. Canker Sores

Entering the maze-like realm of health and recovery, especially for a condition as nettlesome as canker sores, can be an adventure full of uncertainty and agony. MILLIONS of people walk this route, yet it is frequently one of quiet solitude, hidden beneath the shadow of more significant health problems. However, there is a pressing need to conquer this ailment for people who experience the constant sting and sharp of these tiny but powerful mouth sores.

The inspiration for this book began in the peaceful corner of a library, surrounded by tall piles of medical books and periodicals. The pages in front of you are the result of a painstaking compilation of facts, research, and first-hand accounts. Not just another collection of recycled information, the Canker Sore Mastery Bible is a lighthouse that shines through mists of doubt and shows the path to a life free from the pain and suffering caused by canker sores.

How many times have you experienced the first stirrings of a new sore and realised, with a tired acceptance, that the next few days will bring only annoyance and agony? How many times have you searched the web for a cure-all only to be confronted with a deluge of unsubstantiated claims and contradicting guidance? There isn't any such ambiguity in this text. Rather than that, you will find a comprehensive management guide for canker sores—a precisely produced manual that will arm you with knowledge and answer all of your needs.

Although solidly based on science, this method is comprehensive. Like the petals of a healing flower, each chapter opens to disclose the biological causes of canker sores as well as potential environmental and psychological triggers. By giving you, the reader, a thorough grasp of the issue, this book aims to enable you to make informed decisions about your health rather than just listing cures.

When was the last time you enjoyed a meal without the constant fear of pain? Did you ever consider the possibility of having that day come back to you as a new normal rather than just a passing thought? Canker sore management is made easier with the actionable solutions outlined here, which provide you not just the "what" but also the "how." These are tools, refined by the experiences of those who have gone before you and fortified by years of intense study.

Pursuing accessibility, the language used is deliberate and free of the complex medical jargon that frequently causes alienation among those it aims to assist. To ensure that the wisdom contained inside is not ensnared by complexity, clarity and simplicity serve as the guiding principles instead. Each sentence is meant to move you closer to mastery by carefully selecting every word.

Personalized solutions are essential. The management plans that are offered are not uniform because it is crucial to acknowledge the uniqueness of each person. Because they are adaptable, they may be made to fit the particular fabric of your life. Since different people respond differently to different treatments, this book provides a range of options, from conventional medical care to naturally holistic approaches, in recognition of that diversity.

Are you optimistic that you can live a life free of canker sores? When this disease doesn't show any obvious indicators of a smile, is there a day you can picture it? This is where optimism is found, but it's also where a concrete strategy and a set of actions that can lead to that exact result are found.

I encourage you to interact with the material as you turn each page. Ask yourself questions as well as inquiries of the text. Let scepticism work for you and curiosity lead the way. There is an area where comprehension grows and where the seeds of mastery are planted in the conversation between the writer and the reader.

You have a friend, an exemplar, and possibly even comfort in this book. It is the result of many hours of research and the personification of one determined effort: giving you the tools to take charge of your canker sores and get back the quality of life you deserve.

Symptoms and Signs

Setting out on a voyage through the maze-like realm of health and recovery, especially when it comes to a condition as venomous as canker sores, can be unsettling and uncertain. Millions of people walk this journey, but it's frequently done in quiet alone, hidden by the shadow of more serious health problems. However, the fight to overcome this ailment is urgent for people who experience the constant sting and sharp of these little but powerful oral lesions.

This book began in the peaceful corner of a library, surrounded by tall volumes of medical journals and texts. The pages that are in front of you are a carefully curated collection of facts, research, and firsthand accounts. The Canker Sore Mastery Bible is a guide that illuminates the path to a life free from the discomfort of canker sores, not merely a collection of repeated facts.

How often have you experienced the first tingle and realised, with a tired acceptance, that the next few days would be characterised by the discomfort and annoyance of a fresh sore? How often have you searched the internet for a cure-all only to be confronted with a deluge of unsubstantiated claims and contradicting guidance? You won't find any such uncertainty in this book. Rather, you'll find a comprehensive management guide for canker sores that has been painstakingly designed to meet your needs and provide you with information.

This technique is scientifically based but holistic. Like a healing flower's petals, each chapter reveals the biological causes of canker sores as well as potential environmental and psychological triggers. This book aims to provide you, the reader, a thorough understanding of the disease so that you can make educated decisions about your health rather than just listing cures.

When was the last time you enjoyed a meal without the fear of agony hanging over you? Have you ever wished that day might come back to you as the new normal rather than just a passing thought? The techniques outlined here are designed to be practical, giving you the "what" as well as the "how" of managing canker sores. These are instruments, refined by the experiences of those who have gone before you and fortified by years of intense study.

The language used is deliberate and free of the complicated medical jargon that frequently turns off the people it is intended to assist, all in the spirit of accessibility. Rather, simplicity and clarity serve as the guiding principles, making sure that complication does not entangle the wisdom that is present. Each sentence is carefully constructed to move you closer to mastery with every word chosen.

Tailored solutions are essential. Since it is so important to acknowledge individuality, the management plans that are offered are not all-inclusive. They are adjustable and made to fit the particular fabric of your life. This book recognises that everyone has different needs, and it provides a range of options, from naturally holistic to traditional medical approaches.

Do you think it is possible to live a life free of canker sores? When the grin in the mirror is free from the obvious symptoms of this illness, is it possible for you to picture that day? Not only is there hope, but there's also a concrete plan, a set of actions that, if followed, can bring about that exact result.

I want you to actively interact with the material as you turn each page. Pose inquiries to the text and, in turn, to yourself. Give yourself permission to follow your curiosity and use your scepticism to your advantage. Understanding grows and the seeds of mastery are sowed in the discourse between the writer and the reader.

This is your guide, your friend, and maybe even your comfort. It is the result of many hours of research and the personification of one unshakable dedication: giving you the tools to take charge of your canker sores and get back the quality of life you deserve.

The symptoms and signs of canker sores are multifaceted, encompassing a range of indicators that collectively contribute to the clinical presentation of this oral condition. The following key points will be explored in detail:
1. Pain and Discomfort
2. Lesion Characteristics
3. Associated Symptoms
4. Duration and Recurrence

a. Localized pain and discomfort in the oral cavity are a defining feature of canker sores. People frequently describe a stinging, continuous feeling that gets worse when they eat, drink, or talk. Movement of the mouth muscles and contact with food or beverages often exacerbate the discomfort. This particular discomfort can have a major negative effect on a person's quality of life by making it impossible to carry out daily oral tasks and creating a great deal of distress.

a. Canker sores appear as shallow, oval or round lesions with a red border and a white or yellow core. These distinguishing features enable visual inspection-based identification of them, distinguishing them from other oral disorders. Lesions can differ in size; some may show up as tiny, single ulcers, while others may manifest as more extensive or many sores. Furthermore, the fact that these lesions are visible on particular oral mucosa regions—like the tongue, inner cheeks, or gums—helps identify them even more.

c. People with canker sores may also have related symptoms that add to the overall clinical picture, in addition to localised pain and discomfort. Increased sensitivity to hot, spicy, or acidic foods is one of these symptoms, along with a generalised sensation of mouth irritation. Because of the lesions, some people may also report having trouble keeping up with their oral cleanliness, which raises questions about oral hygiene and the risk of developing secondary infections.

d. Canker sores can last for a variety of lengths of time, but most lesions cure in one to two weeks. But one characteristic that sets this illness apart is the recurrence of these mouth ulcers. Over time, people may suffer from canker sores more than once, with differing intervals between episodes. Canker sores are chronic because of their cyclical recurrence pattern, which emphasises how crucial it is to comprehend and treat this element of the illness.

Studies have repeatedly shown that discomfort and suffering are the main signs of canker sores. Research has additionally indicated that the distinctive features of the lesion are repeatable, offering a dependable foundation for medical diagnosis. Further highlighting the importance of these indications are patient testimonials, which frequently highlight the distressing nature of the related symptoms and the impact of recurrent episodes on their everyday life.

Understanding the telltale signs and symptoms of canker sores is essential to enabling prompt intervention and treatment plans. When people recognise that they have canker sores, they can take preventative action to lessen their pain and discomfort. Some proactive measures include applying topical analgesics or changing their diet to reduce irritation. Furthermore, realising that recurrences are cyclical gives people the ability to plan ahead for upcoming episodes, take specific preventive action, and see a professional when necessary.

The thorough explanation of canker sore symptoms and indicators provide a strong basis for the investigation of treatment options that follows. A nuanced approach to canker sore therapy is made possible by an understanding of the clinical appearance of this ailment, which leads readers from recognition to proactive involvement with the concepts of comprehensive care.

Through exploring the nuances of canker sore symptoms and indicators, people get the understanding and intuition required to recognise and manage this difficult oral ailment. The subsequent section of our expedition will explore the complex field of management techniques, enabling readers to take a holistic approach to mastering canker sores.

One characteristic that distinguishes canker sores is localised pain and discomfort in the oral cavity. People often experience a constant, stinging sensation that worsens with food, drink, or conversation. Oral muscle activity and contact with food or drink can often make the irritation worse. This specific discomfort can cause a tremendous deal of distress and make it impossible for a person to perform everyday oral duties, which can have a major negative impact on their quality of life.

a. Canker sores have a white or yellow core and a red border, appearing as shallow, oval or round lesions. These unique characteristics allow for visual inspection-based identification, setting them apart from other oral illnesses. Lesions can vary in size; some may appear as little, isolated sores, while others may take the form of larger, multiple sores. These lesions are further distinguished by the fact that they are evident on certain oral mucosa regions, such as the tongue, inner cheeks, or gums.

c. In addition to localised pain and suffering, people with canker sores may also experience associated symptoms that contribute to the overall clinical picture. One of these symptoms, combined with a widespread feeling of tongue irritation, is an increased sensitivity to hot, spicy, or acidic foods. Some individuals may also have difficulty maintaining proper oral hygiene as a result of the lesions, which raises concerns over oral hygiene practises and the potential for subsequent infections.

d. Although canker sores can heal in a number of ways, most lesions do so in a week or two. But the recurrence of these mouth ulcers sets this condition apart from others. People may experience multiple canker sore episodes throughout time, with varying intervals between them. Because of their cyclical recurrence pattern, canker sores are considered chronic, underscoring the need of understanding and managing this aspect of the illness.

Research has consistently demonstrated that the primary symptoms of canker sores are discomfort and suffering. Studies have also shown that the characteristic characteristics of the lesion are reproducible, providing a reliable basis for medical diagnosis. Patient testimonials, which often emphasise the distressing nature of the associated symptoms and the impact of recurrent episodes on their daily lives, serve as additional evidence of the significance of these indications.

To enable timely intervention and treatment programmes, it is vital to comprehend the unmistakable signs and symptoms of canker sores. People can reduce their pain and anguish by taking preventative measures as soon as they become aware that they have canker sores. Using topical analgesics or altering their diet are two proactive ways to lessen inflammation. In addition, understanding that recurrences are cyclical enables individuals to make plans for impending episodes, implement targeted preventive measures, and seek professional assistance when required.

The in-depth description of canker sore signs and symptoms serves as a solid foundation for the ensuing research into available treatments. Understanding the clinical manifestation of this condition enables readers to take a more nuanced approach to treating canker sores, taking them from recognition to proactive involvement with the concepts of complete care.

Through examining the subtleties of canker sore signs and symptoms, people get the knowledge and intuition needed to identify and treat this challenging oral condition. In order to help readers handle canker sores holistically, we will delve into the intricate realm of management approaches in the next portion of our voyage.

The potential triggers for canker sores span a diverse spectrum, encompassing various factors that have been implicated in the etiology and pathogenesis of these oral ulcers. The following key points will be explored in detail:

1. Dietary Factors
2. Oral Trauma and Mechanical Irritation
3. Stress and Emotional Disturbances
4. Hormonal Fluctuations
5. Immunological Factors
6. Genetic Predisposition

a. The relationship between food ingredients and the emergence of canker sores is a complicated one that needs serious thought. Certain foods have been linked to either causing or aggravating canker sores in those who are vulnerable, including citrus fruits, spicy foods, and acidic drinks. These dietary components' abrasive qualities may cause mucosal damage and mechanical irritation, which will facilitate the development and spread of canker sores.

b. Oral mucosal trauma, resulting from forceful brushing, dental work, or inadvertent biting, can cause canker sores to develop. The development of these mouth ulcers may be accelerated by the physical rupture of the fragile mucosal barrier brought on by mechanical stimulation. In addition, improperly fitted orthodontic equipment or dental appliances can continuously push against the oral tissues, causing persistent discomfort and perhaps leading to the development of canker sores.

c. Emotional problems and psychological stress have been identified as possible canker sore triggers. Because of the complex interactions between the immune system and the central nervous system, immunological responses can become dysregulated, which puts people at risk for developing oral ulcers when under stress. Stress can also lead to the emergence of maladaptive coping mechanisms like bruxism or oral habits, which increase the likelihood of developing canker sores.

d. It has been established that changes in hormones, especially in women, may act as a trigger for canker sores. Changes in hormones during menstruation, pregnancy, or menopause might affect mucosal integrity and immunological function, making people more vulnerable to oral ulcers. Canker sores may arise as a result of the complex hormonal environment, which may regulate inflammatory responses and oral mucosal vulnerability.

e. The pathophysiology of canker sores is significantly influenced by the delicate balance of immune control. These mouth ulcers can develop more quickly if there is a dysregulation of immune responses, which can be brought on by environmental causes, systemic diseases, or genetic predispositions. Immunological variables may increase the susceptibility of oral mucosal tissues to the development of canker sores. These variables include changes in cytokine profiles, immune cell activity, and inflammatory pathways.

f. Canker sore susceptibility has been found to be significantly influenced by genetic predisposition. The occurrence of genetic variants linked to immune system and mucosal integrity, as well as familial clustering, emphasise the inherited aspect of canker sore development. An individual's risk profile for developing recurrent canker sores is further shaped by the interaction of environmental variables and genetic predisposition.

The relationship between dietary triggers, oral trauma, and stress and the development of canker sores has been clarified by epidemiological investigations. Additionally, studies looking at the genetic foundation of canker sores have found particular gene variants and familial patterns that emphasise the condition's hereditary nature. Testimonials from people who experience recurrent canker sores frequently emphasise how stress, certain foods, and oral hygiene practises either cause or worsen their mouth ulcers; these first-hand accounts offer insights into the effects of various triggers.

Knowing the possible causes of canker sores gives people the information they need to put focused prevention measures into place. People can proactively manage their vulnerability to canker sores by recognising and reducing food triggers, maintaining good oral hygiene, and implementing stress-reduction strategies. Furthermore, understanding the impact of hormone fluctuations and genetic predisposition enables people to have knowledgeable conversations with healthcare practitioners and investigate individualised treatment plans catered to their specific risk factors.

Investigating putative canker sore triggers reveals the complex interactions between physiological, genetic, and environmental elements that affect the aetiology of these oral ulcers. This thorough comprehension serves as the basis for the ensuing definition of focused treatment approaches, guiding readers with ease from the explanation of triggers to the application of preventative actions for canker sore mastery.

Through exploring the diverse range of possible causes of canker sores, people can become more adept at identifying the intricate interactions between variables that could hasten the development of these mouth ulcers. Next up on our journey, we'll explore the strategic field of management strategies, giving readers the knowledge and skills they need to take a holistic approach to mastering canker sores.

Canker Sores Vs. Cold Sores

There are two different oral disorders that can bring discomfort and annoyance to persons who have them: canker sores and cold sores. These oral lesions have various etiologies and manifest with different clinical symptoms, although having similar appearances and locations. The purpose of this comparison is to clarify the differences between cold sores and canker sores, providing information on their subtleties and wider consequences for patient education and therapeutic management. This analysis aims to provide people with a thorough understanding of canker sores and cold sores by exploring the minute intricacies of these oral illnesses. This will enable them to make informed decisions and implement preventative treatment techniques.

Aphthous ulcers, another name for canker sores, are painful, recurrent lesions that appear on the oral mucosa, which includes the soft palate, inner surfaces of the lips, cheeks, and tongue. These shallow, round, or oval ulcers have a red, inflamed border around them, while the core is usually white or yellowish. Cold sores, on the other hand, also known as fever blisters or herpes labialis, appear as fluid-filled blisters on and around the lips and are sometimes accompanied by burning, tingling, or itchy feelings. Knowing the differences between cold and canker sores is important for proper diagnosis, treatment, and patient education. It also has potential consequences for public health and disease prevention.

By contrasting canker sores with cold sores, we hope to clarify the key distinctions between these two oral disorders and offer light on their different causes, clinical presentations, and methods of treatment. Through the enumeration of the characteristics that set canker sores and cold sores apart, this comparative analysis seeks to provide patients, healthcare providers, and the general public with the information required to make the distinction between these two entities, thus enabling prompt and focused interventions. Additionally, knowing the distinctive qualities of cold sores and canker sores can provide a more sophisticated understanding of oral mucosal lesions, which may enhance patient outcomes, preventative measures, and public awareness.

The standards used to compare canker and cold sores include a range of factors, such as their etiologies, clinical manifestations, pathophysiological processes, infectiousness, patterns of recurrence, and methods of treatment. By covering these crucial elements, this analysis aims to offer a thorough and impartial perspective on the differences between cold sores and canker sores, making it an invaluable tool for researchers, medical professionals, and anyone who are impacted by these oral illnesses.

Both cold sores and canker sores are lesions that develop in the oral cavity, causing discomfort and lowering the quality of life for the person who gets them. But that is about where the commonalities between these oral disorders stop. Although painful ulcers are a common feature of both canker sores and cold sores, their etiologies differ greatly. As explained in the section above, canker sores are recurrent, non-infectious lesions that can be brought on by a variety of reasons, including food, oral trauma, stress, hormone changes, immunological variables, and genetic susceptibility. On the other hand, most cold sores are caused by HSV-1, a subtype of the herpes simplex virus (HSV). Cold sores are contagious, which sets them apart from canker sores. The virus can spread through asymptomatic shedding or direct contact with active lesions.

Canker sores and cold sores differ not only in their etiologies but also in their clinical manifestations, pathophysiological processes, infectious characteristics, and approaches to therapy. Canker sores are defined by painful, shallow ulcers that have a white or yellowish centre and a red, inflamed border. On and around the lips, cold sores appear as fluid-filled blisters, frequently accompanied by prodromal symptoms like burning, tingling, or stinging. In contrast to cold sores, which are caused by a primary infection or reactivation of the herpes simplex virus, canker sores are caused by local immune dysregulation, mucosal damage, and inflammatory responses. This results in the production of vesicles and subsequent ulceration. Canker sores do not require the same considerations for disease transmission, preventive measures, or antiviral therapy that cold sores do due to their infectious nature.

Making use of visual aids like pictures, charts, or diagrams helps improve comprehension of the differences between cold sores and canker sores. In addition to the textual analysis, visual representations of the clinical presentations, microscopic characteristics, and pathophysiological mechanisms linked to various oral disorders can offer insightful information about their variations, enhancing the reading experience for readers.

A deeper understanding of the heterogeneous character of oral mucosal lesions, including both infectious and non-infectious etiologies, can be gained by contrasting canker sores with cold sores. Healthcare practitioners can improve their diagnostic skills, customise their therapy strategies, and inform patients about the distinct features and consequences of cold sores and canker sores by clarifying the differences between these illnesses. The analysis also highlights the wider implications for disease prevention, patient education, and public health, highlighting the significance of precise diagnosis, focused interventions, and well-informed decision-making in clinical practise and public health campaigns.

Differentiating between canker sores and cold sores is still relevant today when it comes to patient treatment, illness prevention, and public health. Given the frequency of mucosal lesions of the mouth and the possibility of misinterpretation or misdiagnosis, it is critical to distinguish between cold sores and canker sores. A better understanding of the distinct traits, causes, and treatment approaches of canker and cold sores among medical professionals, patients, and the general public can result in better clinical outcomes, raised public awareness, and proactive approaches to illness prevention and patient education.

To sum up, the contrast between cold and canker sores highlights the key differences between the two oral illnesses, providing information about their distinct traits, causes, clinical manifestations, and treatment strategies. Through a thorough examination of the minute details surrounding canker sores and cold sores, this analysis offers a thorough comprehension of these oral lesions, equipping researchers, healthcare providers, and those impacted by these conditions with the knowledge required for precise diagnosis, focused interventions, and well-informed decision-making. Accepting the subtle distinctions between cold sores and canker sores can promote a more sophisticated approach to patient care, public health campaigns, and illness prevention, which will ultimately lead to better clinical results and increased public knowledge of diseases of the oral mucosa.

The Impact on Daily Life

When we explore the world of canker sores, we find that these seemingly benign oral lesions can have a significant effect on a number of daily activities. We will look at how canker sores can impact speech, eating, and general quality of life in this chapter. By dissecting a particular case and outlining the difficulties, approaches, and outcomes, we hope to extract more general lessons and stimulate additional involvement with canker sore care.

Consider Emma, a bright young professional who is committed to advancing her public relations career. She enjoys the fast-paced work atmosphere where she is always interacting with clients, coworkers, and the media. Her canker sores, which present serious obstacles to her everyday activities and general well-being, stifle her excitement. The scene is a busy metropolis, and Emma's way of living matches the fast-paced, high-stakes nature of her line of work.

In this case study, Emma, a 28-year-old public relations executive, is the main character. Her busy schedule and frequent interactions call for confident manner and unambiguous communication. In addition to causing physical suffering, her frequent canker sores have also made her feel self-conscious and frustrated. Emma is receiving support in managing her canker sores from a multidisciplinary team headed by physician and health and fitness coach Dr. Ankita Kashyap. Experts in self-care techniques, psychology, nutrition, and other health and wellness domains make up the team, which takes a multidisciplinary approach to Emma's wellbeing.

Emma faces several challenges as a result of her recurrent canker sores. First of all, she finds it difficult to eat and speak comfortably due to the pain and discomfort caused by the oral lesions. Second, she feels self-conscious and less confident in social situations because of the obvious canker sores on her lips and oral mucosa. Finally, her personal and professional lives are disrupted by the unpredictable nature of canker sore outbreaks, which causes anxiety and irritation. All of these difficulties have a major effect on Emma's general well-being and quality of life.

Emma, along with the multidisciplinary team headed by Dr. Ankita Kashyap, devised a comprehensive plan that included dietary changes, stress management approaches, self-care tactics, and lifestyle modifications to address the challenges presented by recurrent canker sores. Emma got psychological support and individualised treatment to help her deal with the emotional burden of having canker sores. Her diet and nutrition were also adjusted to include foods that lower inflammation and improve oral health. Emma's daily regimen included self-care behaviours like relaxation exercises, oral hygiene, and targeted therapies during outbreaks of canker sores.

After using the multimodal method, Emma saw significant improvements in the way she managed her canker sores. Her episodes became less frequent and less severe, which gave her greater confidence to interact with others and in her professional life. Emma felt more in control and resilient when dealing with canker sores thanks to the pain management and oral discomfort techniques. Moreover, the comprehensive assistance provided by the interdisciplinary team enabled Emma to effectively manage the obstacles presented by her oral lesions, leading to a noticeable improvement in her general quality of life.

Emma's case study provides significant insights into the treatment of this common oral ailment. Emma had recurrent canker sores. It emphasises the value of an all-encompassing, individualised strategy that includes food adjustments, lifestyle adjustments, psychological support, and self-care practises. It also highlights the connections between emotional health, physical symptoms, and work performance, highlighting the necessity of all-encompassing approaches that address the complex effects of canker sores on day-to-day functioning.

Within the framework of this case study, visual aids including illustrations of dental hygiene procedures, nutritional recommendations for dental health, and relaxation methods can enhance comprehension of the all-encompassing strategy used to treat recurrent canker sores. Furthermore, images of Emma's oral lesions before and after can be used to illustrate how the diverse management techniques have affected her health.

Emma's experience with treating recurrent canker sores serves as an example of the more general storey of holistic medicine and wellness promotion that Dr. Ankita Kashyap and her associates support. The case study complies with the main subject of providing people with customised solutions for complete oral health management by tackling the problems caused by canker sores in a multifaceted manner. It emphasises how self-care practises, dietary adjustments, psychological support, and lifestyle changes can all help lessen the impact that canker sores have on day-to-day activities.

Thinking back on Emma's path of transformation in the treatment of her recurrent canker sores, a crucial question is raised: How can the lessons learned from this case study be applied to preventative treatment plans for people with similar oral conditions? This inquiry stimulates more thought and acts as a catalyst for discussing the wider ramifications of managing canker sores holistically. It also encourages research and development in the area of holistic wellness and dental healthcare.

Myth-Busting: Common Misconceptions

: Aphthous ulcers, another name for canker sores, are a common and frequently misdiagnosed oral ailment that affects a sizable section of the population. These painful oral lesions can develop on the soft tissues of the mouth, such as the inner cheeks, lips, tongue, and throat. They are round or oval in shape, with a white or yellow centre and a red border. Canker sores are a common condition, but they're often obscured by myths and misconceptions, which can lead to incorrect perceptions about their causes, treatment, and consequences. To promote a thorough awareness of canker sores and enable efficient management options, it is crucial to debunk these beliefs and present accurate facts. The main problem at hand is the persistence of widespread false perceptions about canker sores, which frequently result in incorrect assumptions and inadequate management strategies. People who are impacted by canker sores often experience uncertainty and bewilderment due to misinformation about the causes, symptoms, and therapies of these oral lesions. This false information also contributes to beliefs regarding canker sores' contagiousness, link to poor dental hygiene, and irreversible effects on day-to-day functioning. Because of this, people who are dealing with canker sores could experience needless anxiety and worry, which makes it more difficult for them to get the help they need and put effective management techniques into practise. The continuation of these false beliefs may have negative consequences for those who are suffering from canker sores. Erroneous assumptions may lead people to pursue unsafe or ineffectual treatments, worsening the pain and delaying the healing of canker sores. Furthermore, the stigma and misconceptions surrounding canker sores can cause affected individuals to feel alone, self-conscious, and anxious, which can negatively impact their emotional health and general quality of life. Furthermore, false beliefs about canker sores that persist in the general public can make it more difficult to provide truthful information and sympathetic assistance to those who are dealing with these oral lesions. A comprehensive strategy that includes education, awareness-raising, and the dissemination of evidence-based information is necessary to address these myths. People can acquire a better awareness of canker sores and be better equipped to make decisions regarding its management by dispelling common misconceptions about the ailment and providing correct information. In order to implement this solution, healthcare professionals, educators, and community activists must work together to disseminate factual information and correct myths via a variety of channels, such as internet forums, public health campaigns, and educational materials. The creation and distribution of educational materials that dispel common misconceptions regarding canker sores constitute the implementation of this approach. These resources ought to clarify the actual reasons behind canker sores, dispel misconceptions about their spread and connection to good oral hygiene, and provide evidence-based treatment recommendations. When it comes to interacting with people who have canker sores, educating them about the condition and encouraging candid conversations to clear up any misunderstandings or worries they may have, healthcare providers are essential. Moreover, community outreach programmes and public health campaigns can help distribute accurate information about canker sores widely, creating a supportive environment for those who are dealing with these oral lesions. By debunking myths and presenting accurate facts regarding canker sores, the anticipated results include a greater knowledge and comprehension of the ailment among those who are impacted as well as the general public. This improved understanding may result in more educated decisions on how to treat canker sores, which may lessen the discomfort and anguish that afflicted patients endure. Furthermore, the development of a precise information base can aid in the de-stigmatization of canker sores by creating a compassionate and encouraging atmosphere that encourages candid discussions and useful management techniques. Although the core of comprehensive management is the suggested technique of debunking myths and supplying accurate information about canker sores, other strategies can support these initiatives. These could include creating specialised support groups for people with canker sores, incorporating teaching about canker sores into oral health curriculum, and working with media organisations to provide correct information to a larger audience. Adopting a comprehensive strategy that incorporates several tactics will strengthen the effort to debunk misconceptions and offer factual information regarding canker sores, creating a nurturing atmosphere for those who are coping with this common oral ailment.

In summary, in order to promote a thorough awareness of canker sores and enable efficient management options, it is critical to provide accurate information and debunk common myths surrounding the condition. People with canker sores can navigate their experiences with more clarity and confidence when common misconceptions are dispelled and evidence-based knowledge is provided, which will eventually improve their quality of life and overall well-being. By working together and implementing focused campaigns, the project to debunk the myths surrounding canker sores can create a welcoming atmosphere that encourages wise choices and gives people the ability to properly treat this common oral ailment.

When to Seek Medical Attention

Before we go into the detailed care of canker sores, let's talk about the crucial part of determining when you should seek expert medical help. Even while canker sores are common and generally not dangerous, there are situations when they require medical attention from qualified doctors. Recognizing the warning indications of a need for medical guidance is essential to prompt intervention and efficient management, which reduces the risk of complications and eases the discomfort of those living with these oral lesions. The main problem at hand is the lack of agreement and clarity surrounding the point at which people with canker sores should seek medical assistance. This uncertainty may cause delayed action, which could exacerbate pain and make it more difficult for canker sores to heal. Furthermore, in the lack of clear standards, people may compromise their dental health and general well-being by seeking medical counsel too soon, spending needless money on healthcare, or failing to recognise warning signs that call for professional action. There might be serious repercussions if the symptoms of canker sores are ignored and medical attention is not sought. Canker sores can worsen, last longer, and take longer to heal if treatment is given too slowly or insufficiently. Additionally, some systemic diseases, such immune system dysfunctions or nutritional deficiencies, can present as canker sore-like oral lesions. In these cases, prompt medical examination is necessary to determine the cause of the disease and create a treatment plan. Those who have canker sores may experience increased emotional anguish, unnecessary discomfort, and possible problems if these warning signs are ignored. The identification of distinct signs that require medical care is crucial in order to tackle this problem. Providing thorough recommendations that explain the particular conditions that call for medical assessment to those afflicted with canker sores can enable them to make educated decisions regarding obtaining medical counsel. In order to provide a systematic framework that identifies the symptoms that require medical treatment, this solution requires the cooperation of healthcare professionals, educators, and people who have canker sores. This will encourage a proactive approach to the management of canker sores. Putting this idea into practise means creating and distributing teaching materials that outline the symptoms of canker sores that require medical attention. These resources ought to offer unambiguous and succinct advice on the telltale signs that demand a professional assessment. These include the extent, duration, and location of canker sores, in addition to any accompanying systemic symptoms that might indicate a medically intervenable underlying condition. Health care providers are essential in helping people with canker sores by educating them about the symptoms that require medical attention and encouraging candid conversations to allay fears and doubts about consulting a specialist. By providing precise guidelines for determining when medical attention is appropriate for canker sores, the anticipated results include an increased level of consciousness and comprehension among those who are impacted, allowing them to make well-informed decisions about seeking professional evaluation when needed. This improved understanding may result in prompt care, which may lessen the length, intensity, and psychological discomfort connected to canker sores. Furthermore, the distribution of organised instructions can help empower those impacted by canker sores by encouraging proactive involvement with their oral health and general well-being. Although the suggested method of identifying distinct signs that require medical intervention for canker sores is the cornerstone of all-encompassing care, other strategies can support these initiatives. These could include the creation of digital applications that offer individualised advice on seeking medical attention for canker sores, the integration of structured assessment tools into healthcare settings to assist people in self-identifying the signs necessitating professional evaluation, and the creation of telemedicine platforms for remote consultation with medical professionals. Adopting a comprehensive strategy that incorporates several tactics can strengthen the effort to enable prompt intervention and efficient treatment of canker sores, therefore improving the welfare of patients suffering from this common oral ailment.

To sum up, the identification of distinct signs that require medical care from a specialist is crucial for promoting an informed and proactive approach to the treatment of canker sores. The endeavour to determine when to seek medical attention for canker sores can reduce the risk of complications, ease emotional distress, and create a supportive environment that encourages proactive engagement with oral health and overall well-being by providing structured guidelines and raising awareness among affected individuals.

The Science Behind Canker Sores

Genetic Factors and Predisposition

Aphthous ulcers, another name for canker sores, are prevalent oral lesions that afflict a large percentage of the population. Numerous studies have been conducted on the aetiology of canker sores, and it is generally accepted that a number of factors play a role in their development. Among these variables, genetic predisposition has become a fascinating field of research, posing fascinating queries on the contribution of genetics to canker sore susceptibility.

The objective of this chapter is to investigate the role that genetic variables play in the susceptibility to canker sores and to clarify the processes that underlie the inherited aspect of this illness.

A substantial amount of evidence backs up the idea that genetics is a major element in the development of canker sores. Research has repeatedly shown that those with a positive family history of canker sores have a higher prevalence of the ailment. Furthermore, a substantial hereditary component in the susceptibility to this ailment has been discovered by twin studies, which show that monozygotic twins had a significantly greater concordance rate for canker sores than dizygotic twins.

Genetic association studies have been used to study the heritability of canker sores. These research have revealed certain genetic markers that have been linked to an increased risk of developing canker sores. The aetiology of canker sores has been linked to differences in genes related to immune regulation and inflammatory pathways. These findings provide insight into the genetic mechanisms behind the vulnerability to this ailment.

Although there is strong evidence that genetic predisposition plays a role in predisposing individuals to canker sores, it is important to recognise that environmental variables may also play a role in conjunction with genetic tendency. In genetically sensitive individuals, environmental stressors such stress, nutrition, and oral trauma can aggravate the development of canker sores, compounding the interaction between environmental and genetic components.

Even with the influence of environmental factors, there is a strong familial aggregation of canker sores, and genetic investigations consistently show that genetic factors play a key role in predisposing individuals to this ailment. The tendency of an individual to acquire canker sores is not solely determined by their genetic predisposition; environmental factors also play a role in moulding this susceptibility.

Population-based studies that have found particular genetic variants linked to an increased risk of developing canker sores provide additional evidence for the genetic basis of canker sores. These results support the complex interaction between the pathophysiological mechanisms underlying the development of canker sores and genetic predisposition.

In conclusion, research on the complex and fascinating topic of how hereditary variables may predispose people to canker sores is needed. From family aggregation to genetic association studies, the evidence for the heritability of canker sores emphasises the important role that genetic variables play in determining a person's vulnerability to this ailment. Canker sores are definitely influenced by environmental variables, but genetic susceptibility to the disorder is still a crucial element. This highlights the need for more research to clarify the complex interactions between genetic and environmental factors in the pathophysiology of canker sores.

Nutritional Deficiencies Linked to Canker Sores

Research on the connection between nutritional inadequacies and canker sores has been particularly interesting since new data points to the possibility that deficiency in some nutrients may have a role in the development and aggravation of these oral lesions. In order to shed insight on the underlying mechanisms and management implications of canker sores, this chapter will examine the compelling correlation between dietary inadequacies and the illness.

This chapter will primarily investigate the claim that certain nutritional inadequacies play a role in the onset and recurrence of canker sores. It is hypothesised that deficits in essential nutrients—like iron, folate, and vitamin B12—may make people more susceptible to developing canker sores. This emphasises how important a healthy diet is to treating this problem.

Canker sores and nutritional inadequacies have been linked in a number of studies, offering strong evidence in favour of this assertion. Studies have consistently shown that those who consume insufficient amounts of vital nutrients—especially iron and vitamin B12—are more likely to develop canker sores. Moreover, studies on the nutritional condition of people who get canker sores frequently have found a strong link between the frequency and intensity of canker sore breakouts and low levels of particular nutrients.

Research has focused on how vitamin B12 deficiency contributes to the aetiology of canker sores, with several studies showing how this nutrient affects the health of the oral mucosa. Because vitamin B12 is essential for DNA synthesis, cell division, and nervous system health, mouth ulcers, particularly canker sores, have been related to vitamin B12 deficiencies. Similarly, low iron and folate intake can interfere with the oral mucosa's natural regeneration and repair processes, making people more prone to developing canker sores.

Even though there is a lot of data linking dietary deficits to canker sores, it's important to recognise any confounding variables that can affect how these oral lesions appear. Environmental factors that cause stress and oral damage might worsen the development of canker sores, making it more difficult to attribute these lesions to dietary deficits alone. Canker sores can also be influenced by the use of specific medications and systemic disorders, thus a thorough evaluation of all contributing variables is necessary.

As a reaction to such counterarguments, it is critical to stress that, although nutritional deficiencies may interact with systemic and environmental factors to cause canker sores, the effects of insufficient nutrient intake on the health of the oral mucosa are well-established. The relevance of treating nutritional deficiencies in the treatment of canker sores is highlighted by the molecular pathways via which particular nutrients influence oral ulceration and the consistent findings across varied populations.

Intervention studies that show the effectiveness of nutritional supplements in lowering the frequency and severity of canker sore breakouts provide more evidence for the link between nutritional deficits and canker sores. In particular, studies looking into the effects of iron and vitamin B12 supplementation have shown observable improvements in the healing of mouth ulcers and a reduction in canker sore recurrence, indicating the therapeutic potential of treating nutritional deficiencies in people who are prone to these lesions.

To sum up, the strong correlation between malnutrition and canker sores highlights how important it is to consume enough nutrients to treat this illness. Although the formation of canker sores is a complex process, there is evidence that some nutritional deficits have an impact on the health of the oral mucosa, which suggests that people who are at risk for canker sores should pay more attention to their nutritional condition. Resolving and correcting these inadequacies may present a viable path toward all-encompassing canker sore care, highlighting the necessity of integrated strategies that incorporate dietary interventions as well as environmental factors.

The Role of Stress and Hormones

In the field of oral health research, the relationship among stress, hormone fluctuations, and canker sores has drawn more and more attention. This chapter aims to clarify the complex relationship between hormonal and psychological factors and the development, worsening, and treatment of canker sores. Through an examination of the physiological processes and clinical data, this investigation seeks to clarify the intricate relationship between stress, hormone changes, and the development of canker sores.

This chapter will focus on the main claim that stress and hormone fluctuations have a significant effect on the onset and progression of canker sores. Hormonal imbalances and elevated stress levels are hypothesised to function as triggers, resulting in the start and continuation of canker sore episodes. This assertion emphasises how crucial it is to understand the dynamic influence of hormonal and psychological factors in the overall care of canker sores.

The complex association between stress, hormone fluctuations, and the frequency of canker sores has been extensively supported by scientific research. There is a favourable association between mouth ulcers and stress levels, as epidemiological research have consistently shown that people experiencing elevated psychological stress have a higher frequency of canker sores. Further research on the hormonal dynamics of menstruation and menopause has revealed significant correlations between hormonal fluctuations and canker sore breakout frequency, highlighting the critical role that hormone oscillations play in oral mucosal health.

The complex interactions between immunological regulation and neuroendocrine pathways highlight the effect of stress on mouth ulcers. Stress hormones like cortisol and catecholamines are released, along with a host of other physiological reactions, when psychological stresses like exams, work-related pressures, and interpersonal disputes are present. These hormonal changes can have significant implications on the immune system, inflammatory processes, and the integrity of the oral mucosa, which can facilitate the development and progression of canker sores. In a similar vein, alterations in immunological response and oral mucosal vulnerability have been linked to the varying levels of progesterone and oestrogen during the menstrual cycle and menopausal phase, which may account for the increased risk of canker sores during these hormonal shifts.

Although there is substantial evidence linking stress and hormone fluctuations to canker sores, it is important to recognise that oral ulceration is a complex condition. The exclusive relationship between psychological and hormonal factors and canker sores can become complicated due to the interaction of environmental factors, dietary habits, and genetic predispositions with stress and hormone dynamics. Furthermore, the diversity of personal stress reactions and hormone profiles emphasises the necessity of thorough evaluations that take into account a range of contributing variables to the development of canker sores.

As a reaction to possible rebuttals, it is important to note that although stress and hormone fluctuations do not contribute exclusively to the pathophysiology of canker sores, there is ample evidence of their significant impact on the health of the oral mucosa. A molecular basis for the observed relationships is provided by the complex interplay of stress hormones, immunological regulation, and oral mucosal vulnerability. This highlights the necessity of integrating psychological and hormonal factors in the holistic care of canker sores.

Clinical treatments that have shown the effectiveness of stress-reduction strategies and hormonal therapy in reducing the frequency and severity of canker sore episodes provide more evidence for the influence of stress and hormone changes on canker sores. By reducing psychological discomfort and regulating stress hormone levels, psychological therapies including mindfulness-based stress reduction and cognitive-behavioral therapy have demonstrated promise in reducing the incidence of canker sore breakouts. Further demonstrating the therapeutic potential of addressing stress and hormonal influences in canker sore management, hormonal therapies targeted at stabilising hormonal imbalances have also shown positive effects on lowering the incidence of oral ulcers, especially in individuals with menstruation-related canker sores.

In summary, the complex interactions among stress, hormone fluctuations, and canker sores highlight the complexity of this oral disease and the critical need for all-encompassing treatment approaches. Although there are many factors that contribute to the development of canker sores, the strong evidence that stress and hormonal dynamics have a significant impact on oral mucosal health highlights how important it is to incorporate psychological and hormonal factors into the comprehensive management of canker sores. Personalized canker sore management may be possible by addressing stress and hormone imbalances; this emphasises the need for customised strategies that take psychological, hormonal, and environmental factors into account.

Immunological Aspects

Knowing the immunological components of canker sores is essential to understanding the complex processes that underlie the onset and treatment of this recurrent oral ailment. This chapter explores the intricate immunological mechanisms influencing the development, course, and resolution of canker sores, illuminating the critical role that immune responses play in oral ulceration.

The main argument that will be discussed in this chapter is the immune system's important role in the pathophysiology of canker sores. It is suggested that immune response dysregulation, including both adaptive and innate immunity, contributes significantly to the start and continuation of episodes of canker sores. This assertion highlights how crucial it is to understand the immunological causes of canker sores in order to design focused therapy approaches.

Numerous studies have confirmed the complex relationship between immunological dysregulation and the development of canker sores. Research has demonstrated that the oral mucosa of patients with canker sores has abnormalities in immune cell populations, cytokine profiles, and immune signalling pathways. These findings highlight the critical role that immunological dysfunction plays in the pathophysiology of this illness. Additionally, studies examining genetic predispositions have revealed correlations between particular immune-related gene variants and a heightened vulnerability to canker sores, underscoring the role of the genetic-immune nexus in the genesis of this oral disease.

The complex interactions between inflammatory mediators, immune cell activation, and tissue destruction within the oral mucosa highlight the role that immunological dysregulation plays in canker sores. An imbalance between pro- and anti-inflammatory cytokines is a sign of dysregulated immune responses, which can lead to the development of canker sores in a favourable milieu. Furthermore, immunological reactivity against oral mucosal antigens may be increased as a result of immune surveillance and tolerance mechanism disruptions, which could ultimately result in the development of ulcerative lesions. The fact that immune cells such dendritic cells, T lymphocytes, and natural killer cells are involved in directing the immune responses in canker sore lesions highlights the complex immunological basis of this illness.

Even though there is strong evidence linking immunological dysregulation to canker sores, it is important to recognise that oral ulceration is a complex condition. Canker sores cannot be solely attributed to immunological factors due to the intersection of immune dysregulation with environmental triggers, microbiological effects, and oral mucosal damage. Furthermore, because immune responses vary widely across individuals and because immunological interactions are dynamic, thorough evaluations that take into account a variety of contributing variables to the development of canker sores are required.

In response to possible rebuttals, it is important to stress that, despite immunological dysregulation's significant impact on oral mucosal health being well-documented, it does not operate alone in the pathogenesis of canker sores. A molecular basis for the observed relationships is provided by the complex interplay among immune mediators, cellular responses, and tissue homeostasis, highlighting the necessity of incorporating immunological considerations into the comprehensive care of canker sores.

Clinical trials that show the effectiveness of immunomodulatory therapy in reducing the frequency and severity of canker sore episodes provide more evidence for the role of immunological dysregulation in canker sores. By reducing local inflammation and immunological hyperreactivity, targeted therapies such topical corticosteroids and immunomodulatory drugs have demonstrated potential in reducing canker sore outbreaks. Further demonstrating the complex interactions between immune, microbial, and environmental factors in the pathophysiology of this condition, studies on the impact of microbial dysbiosis on immune homeostasis within the oral cavity have also revealed possible connections between microbial imbalances and the aggravation of canker sores.

Finally, the critical role that immunological dysregulation plays in the onset and progression of canker sores highlights the complexity of this oral disease and the critical need for all-encompassing treatment approaches. Although there are many factors that contribute to the formation of canker sores, the strong evidence that immune responses have a significant impact on oral mucosal health highlights how important it is to incorporate immunological considerations into the comprehensive management of canker sores. Personalized canker sore care may be possible by addressing immune dysregulation, which emphasises the need for specialised strategies that take into account immunological, environmental, and microbiological factors.

Epidemiology: Who Gets Canker Sores?

Gaining knowledge of the prevalence and distribution of canker sores in various groups requires an understanding of the epidemiology of this oral ailment. This chapter seeks to clarify the demographic and geographic distribution of canker sore incidence, illuminating the variables affecting the vulnerability to and appearance of this recurrent oral ailment.

The main hypothesis that will be investigated in this chapter concerns the regional and demographic factors that influence the occurrence of canker sores. It is proposed that the epidemiological landscape of canker sores is shaped in large part by age, gender, ethnicity, and geography, which in turn affects the probability that an individual will develop recurrent oral ulceration. This assertion emphasises how crucial it is to identify the demographic and regional variables influencing the prevalence and cost of canker sores in order to develop individualised treatment plans and focused public health initiatives.

A significant amount of information about the frequency and distribution of canker sores in various groups has been made available by epidemiological studies. There is a wide range of reported prevalence rates; estimates show that about 20 percent of the general population is recurrently affected by canker sores. Moreover, studies examining age-related trends have revealed that younger people have a greater incidence of canker sores, with teenagers and young adults being the most afflicted age groups. There is evidence of a gender difference in the incidence of canker sores, with women more likely than men to experience these mouth ulcers. Furthermore, variations in the incidence of canker sores among various ethnic groups have been noted, with some cultures demonstrating a higher vulnerability to recurring mouth ulcers.

Younger people are more susceptible to oral mucosal injuries and have heightened immunological reactivity, which underlies the age-related predisposition for canker sores and increases the frequency of canker sore episodes. Oral hygiene habits, hormonal changes, and genetic predispositions that make women more likely to experience recurring oral ulcerations could all contribute to gender differences in the occurrence of canker sores. Furthermore, the noted ethnic differences in the incidence of canker sores could be a reflection of genetic predispositions, customary eating practises, and oral microbiota compositions that affect how oral ulcers appear in particular cultures.

Although the research that has been presented highlights the demographic and geographic factors that determine the occurrence of canker sores, it is crucial to take into account the potential impact of confounding variables and methodological constraints when conducting epidemiological studies. There is a possibility that the stated prevalence rates across various groups contain biases and inaccuracies due to variations in canker sore reporting and diagnosis, variations in healthcare-seeking behaviours, and discrepancies in access to oral healthcare services. To further identify the true underlying patterns of canker sore recurrence, a sophisticated interpretation of the epidemiological data is required due to the dynamic nature of demographic transitions, lifestyle changes, and environmental factors.

To address such rebuttals, it is imperative to emphasise the strength of the epidemiological data clarifying the regional and demographic factors influencing the occurrence of canker sores. The consistent trends identified across numerous studies and populations verify the influence of age, gender, ethnicity, and geographic location on the epidemiology of canker sores, despite the methodological limitations inherent in epidemiological research. Error-free study designs and thorough data analysis can further improve the accuracy and dependability of epidemiological findings by addressing confounding variables and methodological limitations.

Longitudinal cohort studies that have identified age-specific incidence rates and temporal trends in canker sore occurrence provide additional support for the demographic and geographic factors influencing canker sore prevalence. Furthermore, studies on the geographical distribution of canker sores have revealed differences in the prevalence and burden of the condition in various areas, with food habits, oral hygiene practises, and environmental factors all playing a role in the reported discrepancies. The impact of socioeconomic status, healthcare resource accessibility, and cultural factors on the epidemiology of canker sores highlights the complex relationship between demographic and geographic factors and mouth ulceration.

To sum up, the epidemiological terrain surrounding canker sores is significantly influenced by demographic and geographic factors, which include age, gender, ethnicity, and place of residence. Strong data from epidemiological research emphasises how important it is to map out the frequency and distribution of canker sores across various communities in order to design customised management strategies and focused public health campaigns. Healthcare practitioners and policymakers can improve the comprehensive management of canker sores in communities and populations by developing tailored solutions to reduce the burden of recurring mouth ulcers by understanding the demographic and geographic factors on canker sore incidence.

Current Research and Developments

The rising prevalence and impact on oral health of canker sores, also known as aphthous ulcers, have drawn attention to the research of these ulcers in recent years. Recurrent, excruciating ulcers that damage the oral mucosa, causing pain and compromising oral functioning are known as canker sores. It is clear from reading through the most recent scientific studies and possible discoveries that more study is needed to fully understand the underlying mechanisms, risk factors, and possible treatments for canker sores, a frequent oral ailment.

The earliest known accounts of canker sore-like oral ulcers come from ancient civilizations, including Greek, Roman, and Egyptian medical literature. These early accounts outlined the distinctive characteristics of canker sores and made an effort to offer etiological reasons; frequently, they blamed the ulcers on abnormalities in dental hygiene habits or imbalances in body humours. The historical narratives surrounding canker sores offer fascinating insights into the persistent nature of this oral ailment and its widespread influence on human health throughout many cultural and historical contexts.

- The 19th century saw the development of comprehensive clinical descriptions of canker sores, in which physicians described the clinical characteristics and ulcer's natural progression. Significant developments in clinical observation and documentation provided the foundation for further research endeavours aimed at determining the cause and mechanism of canker sores. An important advancement in our knowledge of canker sores was the clarification of the immune system's function in mediating oral mucosal inflammation and ulceration. The attention has shifted towards immunopathogenic mechanisms underlying the pathogenesis of canker sores as a result of groundbreaking studies that found immunological dysregulations and aberrations that contribute to the formation of recurrent mouth ulcers. - A paradigm change in understanding the genetic susceptibilities and molecular pathways related to the development of canker sores was brought about by the advancement of molecular and genetic studies. Research on the genetics of canker sores revealed polymorphisms in inflammatory cytokine genes and correlations with particular human leukocyte antigen (HLA) alleles, which provided insight into the genetic factors influencing canker sore vulnerability.

- In an effort to identify the complex aetiology of canker sores, there has been a notable increase in interdisciplinary research efforts in recent years that span genetics, immunology, microbiology, and oral medicine. Technological developments in precision medicine, bioinformatics, and high-throughput sequencing have made it easier to conduct thorough investigations into the host immune system, the oral microbiota, and the molecular pathways underlying the pathophysiology of canker sores.

This part could contain graphical representations of the immunological and genetic systems involved in the development of canker sores, scientific illustrations of the pathophysiology of canker sores, or visual reproductions of historical sources. The historical turning points and technological advances in the study of canker sores are better understood with the help of these visual aids.

There are documented cultural and regional differences in the occurrence and treatment of canker sores, highlighting the complex interactions between genetic predispositions, dental hygiene routines, and food habits. Notably, several cultural dietary practices—like consuming hot or acidic foods—have been connected to a higher risk of developing canker sores in particular communities. Furthermore, the observed cultural disparities in canker sore prevalence and severity are partly explained by changes in immunological reactivity and oral microbial assemblages among various ethnic groups.

Research efforts in the present have focused on combining cutting edge molecular and genomic techniques to clarify the complex interactions among genetic predispositions, immunological dysregulations, and microbiological triggers in the pathogenesis of canker sores. Personalized genomic profiling and targeted immunomodulatory medications are two examples of precision medicine principles that could be applied to provide patients with recurrent canker sores with customised therapy plans.

The ongoing debates about the exact aetiology and triggers of canker sores represent one of the major turning points in the history of canker sore research. Although genetic predispositions and immunological dysregulations have been linked to the aetiology of canker sores, the precise interactions between oral microbiota, environmental triggers, and host variables are still being discussed and studied in great detail in scientific research. Moreover, the conversion of scientific discoveries into efficacious therapeutic approaches for canker sores remains a persistent obstacle, requiring coordinated endeavours to close the gap between research outcomes and clinical implementations.

The intersection of historical viewpoints, contemporary scientific discoveries, and developing issues provides a thorough overview of the changing field of canker sore comprehension as we go deeper into the subject. This tour through the history of canker sore mastery is evidence of the ongoing efforts to decipher the mysterious nature of this recurrent oral ailment and to develop novel approaches for its all-encompassing treatment.

Medical Treatments for Canker Sores

Topical Medications: Types and Usage

Introduction to the List:

Topical medicines are important in the management of canker sores because they aid in both pain reduction and healing. The several topical therapies for canker sores, along with their active substances and application techniques, will be thoroughly covered in this section. For those looking to effectively manage canker sores, it is essential to comprehend the many sorts of topical drugs and how to use them.

Presentation of the List:

1. Benzocaine-based Topical Medications
2. Hydrogen Peroxide Rinses
3. Corticosteroid Ointments
4. Topical Antiseptics
5. Herbal and Natural Remedies

Point Elaboration:

Benzocaine-based Topical Medications

a. An Introduction to Benzocaine

A common component of many over-the-counter topical treatments intended to reduce the discomfort caused by canker sores is benzocaine, a local anaesthetic. Its mode of action is to temporarily relieve pain and discomfort by obstructing nerve signals in the body.

b. Application and Mechanism of Action

Benzocaine reduces the feeling of pain and discomfort by numbing the nerve endings when given topically to the affected area. It can be used in a variety of ways depending on personal preferences because it comes in several forms, such as gels, sprays, and lozenges.

c. Proof and Testimonies

Research has indicated that benzocaine-based topical medicines are effective in quickly relieving pain for those with canker sores.

Furthermore, customer testimonies have demonstrated how well benzocaine works to relieve canker sore symptoms.

d. Real-World Uses

Benzocaine-based topical treatments should be used practically by carefully according to the manufacturer's instructions. To avoid any negative effects, users should apply the drug immediately to the affected area, making sure not to exceed the authorised amount.

Rinses with Hydrogen Peroxide

a. Overview of Hydrogen Peroxide

A common mild antiseptic for wound care and mouth hygiene is hydrogen peroxide. It can aid in the cleaning and healing of the canker sore affected region when used as a mouth rinse.

b. Application and Mechanism of Action

By dissolving debris and lowering the bacterial load surrounding the canker sore, hydrogen peroxide's bubbling action promotes healing. For best results, the fluid must be diluted correctly and swished about the mouth.

c. Proof and Testimonies

Research studies have indicated that the use of hydrogen peroxide rinses can aid in reducing the duration and severity of canker sores. Furthermore, anecdotal evidence from individuals who have incorporated hydrogen peroxide rinses into their oral care routine supports its potential benefits in canker sore management.

d. Practical Applications

Before using the hydrogen peroxide solution as a mouthwash, people should dilute it according to the suggested ratio. To prevent potential irritation of oral tissues, users should take care not to swallow the solution and should follow the recommended frequency of usage.

Corticosteroid Ointments

a. Corticosteroids: An Overview

Anti-inflammatory substances found in corticosteroid ointments can aid in lowering canker sore-related swelling, discomfort, and irritation. These drugs are applied directly to the affected area and are usually available with a prescription.

b. Mechanism of Action and Application

By suppressing the immunological response in the affected area, corticosteroids' anti-inflammatory qualities help to lessen the symptoms of canker sores. Using a cotton swab, apply a thin coating of the ointment to the canker sore in a gentle and uniform manner.

c. Evidence and Testimonials

Clinical studies have shown that corticosteroid ointments are effective at hastening the healing of canker sores and relieving pain that is related with them. These results have been supported by the testimonies of people who have used corticosteroid ointments, who highlighted the beneficial effects on their general quality of life.

d. Practical Applications

When using corticosteroid ointments, patients should strictly adhere to their doctor's instructions. It is crucial to take the prescription as prescribed, to keep an eye out for any possible adverse effects, and to notify the prescribing doctor of any concerns.

Topical Antiseptics

a. Topical Antiseptics: An Overview

Topical antiseptics, such chlorhexidine gluconate, work to remove bacteria from the afflicted area and create a conducive environment for canker sore healing.

b. Mechanism of Action and Application

Topical medications possess antiseptic characteristics that hinder the growth of bacteria and fungus, hence averting subsequent infections and promoting the body's inherent healing mechanism. The antiseptic solution is applied by gently swabbing the afflicted region.

c. Evidence and Testimonials

Research has demonstrated how topical antiseptics can help people with canker sores lower their chance of developing secondary infections. User testimonials highlight these topical agents' calming and purifying properties, which enhance comfort during the healing process.

d. Practical Applications

When using topical antiseptics, people should follow the application frequency and duration advised by the manufacturer or their healthcare professional. To keep the antiseptic solution effective, it must be handled and stored properly.

Herbal and Natural Remedies

a. Herbal and Natural Remedies: An Overview

A variety of herbal and natural therapies have been investigated for their potential in controlling canker sores in addition to conventional drugs. These treatments frequently make use of natural substances' anti-inflammatory, antibacterial, and wound-healing capabilities.

b. Mechanism of Action and Application

Ingredients with calming and restorative qualities like licorice, aloe vera, and chamomile may be found in herbal and natural therapies. There are several ways to apply products; they can be applied topically or taken orally as supplements or teas.

c. Evidence and Testimonials

Anecdotal accounts and historic usage patterns have prompted interest in the possible benefits of herbal and natural therapies for canker sore therapy, despite the lack of scientific data to support their efficacy. Using these natural solutions has helped many people find relief and speed up their recovery process.

d. Practical Applications

People who are interested in investigating herbal and natural cures should proceed with caution and speak with a medical practitioner first, especially if they are taking medication or have pre-existing medical concerns. Assuring safety and effectiveness requires sourcing high-quality materials and following prescribed dosages.

Seamless Transitions:

It is clear from our exploration of the wide range of topical treatments available for the treatment of canker sores that each choice has advantages and disadvantages of its own. By being aware of the methods of action, empirical data, and useful applications of these topical treatments, people are better equipped to make judgments about how to manage canker sore symptoms and encourage recovery. We will go deeper into complimentary techniques and holistic strategies in the upcoming sections to fully address the complex nature of managing canker sores.

Oral Medications: A Deeper Dive

Introduction to the List:

Oral medicines are frequently used to treat the symptoms and speed up the healing process in more severe cases of canker sores. Due to the intricacies of oral treatments for canker sores, a thorough comprehension of their actions, possible adverse effects, and contraindications is important. In order to give readers a thorough understanding of the pharmacological profiles and therapeutic uses of the oral drugs frequently used in the treatment of severe canker sores, this section will go into great detail.

Presentation of the List:

1. Systemic Corticosteroids
2. Tetracycline Antibiotics
3. Oral Analgesics
4. Immunomodulatory Agents
5. Vitamin and Mineral Supplements

Point Elaboration:

Systemic Corticosteroids

a. Corticosteroids in Canker Sore Management

Prednisone and dexamethasone are examples of systemic corticosteroids, which are strong anti-inflammatory drugs that act on the entire body. These drugs are usually used orally in the form of tablets or solutions when prescribed for severe canker sores.

b. Mechanism of Action and Application

Systemic corticosteroids work by modifying the immune system, which lowers inflammation and inhibits immunological-mediated mechanisms that lead to the formation of canker sores. Systemic distribution is ensured by oral delivery, which reaches the impacted mucosal surfaces.

c. Evidence and Testimonials

Systemic corticosteroids have been shown through clinical trials to be effective in reducing symptoms and accelerating the healing of severe canker sores. Testimonials from patients have highlighted the significant alleviation and quicker recovery that occurred after starting systemic corticosteroid treatment.

d. Practical Applications

Systemic corticosteroid administration requires careful observation and strict adherence to the recommended dosage and time. Potential side effects, such as immunosuppression and adrenal insufficiency, should be explained to patients and managed carefully under medical supervision.

Tetracycline Antibiotics

a. Role of Tetracyclines in Canker Sore Treatment

Tetracycline antibiotics—like minocycline and doxycycline—have shown promise as treatment for severe canker sores, especially when there may be concurrent bacterial involvement.

b. Mechanism of Action and Application

Tetracyclines' antibacterial qualities work against harmful germs that can worsen canker sore symptoms or slow down the healing process. By ensuring systemic distribution through oral dosing, possible bacterial etiologies that increase the severity of canker sores are addressed.

c. Evidence and Testimonials

In the context of managing canker sores, research studies have clarified the antibacterial efficiency of tetracycline antibiotics, emphasising their function in reducing bacterial burden and encouraging mucosal healing. Testimonials from patients receiving antimicrobial therapy with tetracycline have confirmed the beneficial effects on symptom relief and recuperation.

d. Practical Applications

Patients who are administered antibiotics containing tetracycline ought to follow the suggested dosage, frequency, and course of therapy. Because of possible adverse effects like gastrointestinal problems and photosensitivity, it's crucial to use this medication carefully and under medical supervision.

Oral Analgesics

a. Utilizing Oral Analgesics for Symptomatic Relief

Oral analgesics, such as acetaminophen and nonsteroidal anti-inflammatory medications (NSAIDs), are used to treat severe canker sores and reduce pain and discomfort, improving the quality of life for those who have them.

b. Mechanism of Action and Application

Through the pharmacological modulation of pain signalling pathways and the decrease of inflammatory mediators, oral analgesics are able to lessen subjective pain and discomfort. Targeted alleviation and systemic dispersion are guaranteed by oral administration.

c. Evidence and Testimonials

Clinical data demonstrates the effectiveness of oral analgesics in relieving the symptoms of severe canker sores and increasing the patient's tolerance for the pain that goes along with them. Patient testimonials demonstrate how using oral analgesics has tangibly improved everyday functioning and well-being.

d. Practical Applications

When using oral analgesics, patients should follow the suggested dosages and usage guidelines, keeping in mind possible side effects include gastrointestinal irritation and renal toxicity. Supervision of healthcare is essential, particularly for those with concurrent medication regimens or chronic medical issues.

Immunomodulatory Agents

a. Immune Modulation in Severe Canker Sore Cases

Colchicine and thalidomide are two examples of immunomodulatory medications that are used to control the immune system in cases with severe canker sores in an effort to reduce inflammatory processes and promote healing.

b. Mechanism of Action and Application

These substances have immunomodulatory qualities that control immune cell activity and cytokine production, which reduce inflammation and promote tissue healing in the oral mucosa. The systemic treatment of these medications targets the complex immunological dysregulation that is responsible for severe canker sores.

c. Evidence and Testimonials

Clinical studies have outlined these drugs' immunomodulatory potential in reducing severe canker sore symptoms and accelerating mucosal healing. Testimonies from patients receiving immunomodulatory therapy have demonstrated how immune modulation significantly relieves symptoms and restores oral function.

d. Practical Applications

Immunomodulatory drug use requires close observation for any side effects, such as hematologic irregularities or, in the case of thalidomide, teratogenicity. Before starting therapy, patients should have thorough counselling and go through a rigorous risk assessment.

Vitamin and Mineral Supplements

a. Nutritional Support for the Treatment of Severe Canker Sores

In the case of severe canker sores, vitamin and mineral supplements, especially those containing iron, folate, and B vitamins, are crucial for treating nutritional deficiencies and supporting mucosal healing.

b. Application and Mechanism of Action

These supplements address underlying inadequacies that may worsen severe canker sore symptoms by supporting immune system function, cellular metabolism, and tissue repair. By ensuring systemic circulation, oral administration maximises the nutritional environment for mucosal healing.

c. Proof and Testimonies

Clinical observations have demonstrated how vitamin and mineral supplements can speed up the healing process and lessen the intensity of severe canker sores, especially in those with known dietary deficiencies. Patients who are receiving supplements have attested to the noticeable enhancements in their general health and oral health.

d. Real-World Uses

Individual nutritional status and any drug interactions should be taken into account when choosing and prescribing vitamin and mineral supplements for patients. To evaluate the effectiveness of treatment and guarantee safety, regular monitoring of nutritional indicators is essential.

Seamless Transitions:

It is clear from our exploration of the field of oral drugs for the treatment of severe canker sores that each therapeutic approach has unique advantages and factors to take into account while managing the intricate interaction between symptoms and underlying pathophysiology. Improving the reader's understanding of the pharmacological nuances, clinical data, and practical consequences of these oral therapies facilitates collaborative participation in the management of severe canker sores and empowers informed decision-making. We will go deeper into complementary modalities and integrated approaches in the next sections to fully address the complex aspects of managing severe canker sores.

Corticosteroid Treatments: Pros and Cons

Introduction to the Context:

Since corticosteroids have strong anti-inflammatory qualities and may help reduce the amount of pain associated with these mucosal lesions, their use as a therapy option has attracted a lot of attention in the field of canker sore care. The purpose of this section is to objectively analyse the use of corticosteroids in the management of canker sores by exploring their effectiveness, safety profile, and the complex factors that support their use.

Defining the Problem:

Phthous ulcers, another name for canker sores, are a common oral mucosal ailment that cause painful, spherical or oval lesions on the tongue, buccal mucosa, and other intraoral surfaces. Effective management options are essential due to the recurrent nature of canker sores and their significant impact on oral function and quality of life. Treating the inflammatory cascade and immunological dysregulation that underlie the pathophysiology of canker sores is a challenge, requiring focused therapies to reduce symptoms and hasten the repair of the mucosa.

Highlighting the Consequences:

When canker sores are left untreated, the afflicted person may experience severe side effects such as excruciating pain, poor taste, difficulty speaking, and increased vulnerability to recurrent infections. Moreover, the recurrent nature of canker sores contributes to psychological distress and lowers general well-being, highlighting the necessity of comprehensive management approaches to reduce the severity of these outcomes.

Introducing the Solution(s):

Given their well-known anti-inflammatory and immunosuppressive qualities, corticosteroids present a promising treatment option for the inflammatory basis of canker sores. As corticosteroids have the capacity to regulate immune responses and suppress mucosal inflammation, they offer a potentially effective means of reducing canker sore symptoms and hastening their healing process, which in turn lessens the associated effects on oral health and quality of life.

Detailing the Implementation:

Choosing the right formulations, doses, and treatment durations based on the severity and clinical context of each case is an important part of using corticosteroid therapies wisely in the management of canker sores. Topical corticosteroids, such as fluocinonide or triamcinolone acetonide, can be used to directly target the afflicted mucosal surfaces in oral mucosal applications, but systemic corticosteroids should only be administered under intensive medical supervision in severe cases.

Showcasing Past or Predicted Outcomes:

The benefits of corticosteroid therapies for the management of canker sores have been demonstrated by clinical studies and empirical data. These results include significant pain and discomfort relief, quicker healing of mucosal lesions, and an overall improvement in oral health and function for those who are impacted. Expectations arising from the prudent application of corticosteroids suggest a palpable decrease in the load of symptoms and an expedited course toward mucosal healing, which in turn lessens the subsequent impact of canker sores on the day-to-day activities of persons.

Discussing Alternative Solutions (optional):

Even though corticosteroids are a strong treatment option for canker sores, investigating additional therapeutic approaches is important. Adjunctive tactics, such as dietary changes, immunomodulatory drugs, and mucosal protectants, can be used in addition to or instead of corticosteroid therapies to accommodate a range of clinical presentations and individual responses to different therapeutic methods.

In-depth Examination of Corticosteroid Treatments in Canker Sore Management:

Corticosteroids in the Context of Canker Sore Management:

Systemic and topical corticosteroids have attracted a lot of interest in the treatment of canker sores because of their diverse pharmacological characteristics and ability to alter the inflammatory cascade that drives the development of these mucosal lesions. The fact that corticosteroids are classified as glucocorticoids emphasises their ability to have strong anti-inflammatory, immunosuppressive, and vasoconstrictive actions, which address the classic symptoms of canker sores and promote mucosal healing.

Mechanism of Action and Application:

Corticosteroids work by modifying immune responses, reducing inflammatory mediators, and preventing mucosal inflammation from recurring. This is how they work in the management of canker sores. When used topically, corticosteroids make direct contact with the impacted mucosal surfaces, causing localised reductions in inflammation and aiding in the healing of mucosal lesions. On the other hand, systemic corticosteroid administration results in a more comprehensive immunomodulatory effect, affecting immune responses throughout the body and reducing the inflammatory environment that contributes to the pathophysiology of canker sores.

Efficacy and Safety Profile:

Empirical research and clinical studies have demonstrated the effectiveness of corticosteroid therapies in reducing the severity of symptoms and hastening the healing of canker sores. Notably, topical corticosteroids have proven to be effective in reducing the amount of mucosal involvement, speeding up the healing process, and reducing pain and suffering. Systemic corticosteroids used sparingly have proven to be quite effective in treating severe, refractory canker sores, providing significant comfort and accelerating the mucosal healing process.

Simultaneously, concerns regarding the safety profile of corticosteroid therapies demand careful evaluation. These concerns include possible adverse effects such mucosal atrophy, systemic immunosuppression, and the possibility of candidiasis when using the medication for an extended period of time. Appropriate formulations, dosages, and treatment durations must be carefully chosen, and patients must get constant medical monitoring to minimise side effects and guarantee the best possible outcomes from corticosteroid therapies.

Practical Applications and Considerations:

In order to effectively manage canker sores, corticosteroid therapies require a thorough grasp of their pharmacological profiles, clinical indications, and the subtle factors that support their use. By selecting corticosteroid formulations based on the severity and clinical context of each particular case and carefully adhering to recommended dosages and treatment schedules, one can minimise potential side effects and create an environment that is best for therapeutic outcomes.

Including corticosteroid treatments in a holistic management strategy for canker sores requires easy cooperation between medical professionals and patients. This cooperation includes thorough counselling, careful monitoring for response to treatment, and wise modification of treatment plans in response to clinical progress. Moreover, factors such as possible contraindications, medication interactions, and patient reaction to corticosteroid treatments reinforce the need for customised, patient-centered methods that give priority to safety and effectiveness in the treatment of canker sores.

Given the complex nature of canker sores and the range of clinical presentations that afflict impacted patients, healthcare professionals can better address the inflammatory aetiology of canker sores and create an environment that promotes faster mucosal healing by carefully integrating corticosteroid treatments into a comprehensive treatment plan. This can reduce the burden of symptoms and lessen the subsequent effects on oral health and function.

Conclusion:

The intricate relationship among inflammatory cascades, immunological dysregulation, and mucosal healing highlights the need for focused therapies in the treatment of canker sores, with the goal of reducing the burden of symptoms and accelerating mucosal healing. Because of their strong anti-inflammatory and immunosuppressive qualities, corticosteroid therapies have become a very attractive option for treating the inflammatory basis of canker sores. They provide significant comfort and accelerate the process of mucosal healing.

This critical analysis of corticosteroid treatments for canker sores highlights the need for a prudent, patient-centered approach that balances risk mitigation with optimal therapeutic outcomes. It also covers the treatments' mechanism of action, clinical efficacy, safety profile, and practical considerations. When corticosteroid treatments are smoothly incorporated into a holistic management approach and are combined with supplemental techniques and customised interventions, patients are better equipped to make educated decisions and work together to manage canker sores, which in turn lessens the impact the sores have on oral health and function.

Pain Management Strategies

Relieving pain and improving the quality of life for those who have these recurrent oral mucosal lesions is the main objective of canker sore pain management techniques. Through offering useful tips and direction on how to effectively manage the discomfort associated with canker sores, the goal is to provide readers with an extensive toolkit for reducing the burden of symptoms and creating an atmosphere that promotes quicker mucosal healing.

It is imperative that readers have a basic understanding of the pathophysiology of canker sores, including their origin, clinical symptoms, and the inflammatory mechanisms behind their pathogenesis, before beginning to implement pain management techniques. Moreover, a thorough understanding of the pharmacological characteristics and clinical implications related to pain management modalities—including over-the-counter medications, prescription drugs, and adjunctive therapy—is essential for making educated decisions and developing customised treatment plans.

Depending on the intensity and specific clinical circumstances of each case, pain management strategies for canker sores take a multimodal approach that includes over-the-counter medications, prescription opioids, and complementary therapy modalities. The primary goals are to reduce oral functional impairment, relieve pain and suffering, and hasten mucosal healing in order to lessen the overall burden of canker sores on people's everyday lives.

The step-by-step guide to pain management tactics begins with an explanation of over-the-counter medications, which include topical analgesics, oral analgesic rinses, and barrier protection agents. These medications are intended to alleviate pain, encourage mucosal healing, and reduce irritation. The distinction between prescribed analgesics, corticosteroids, and nonsteroidal anti-inflammatory medicines (NSAIDs) then incorporates a customised strategy to relieve pain and discomfort while targeting the inflammatory basis of canker sores. Additionally, incorporating adjuvant therapy modalities—such as dietary supplements, stress reduction methods, and mucosal protectants—improves the overall pain management strategy and creates an atmosphere that promotes quicker mucosal healing.

When using pain management techniques for canker sores, it's critical to follow recommended dosages and treatment schedules, give careful thought to safety issues, and keep a close eye on treatment response. Furthermore, the necessity for the best possible therapeutic results and improved general well-being is supported by the prudent selection of pain management modalities suited to the severity and clinical context of individual cases, as well as thorough counselling and cooperative engagement with healthcare providers.

The validation of efficacious pain management techniques for canker sores depends on the significant reduction of pain and discomfort, the prompt healing of mucosal lesions, and the general improvement of oral function and patient satisfaction. Through careful observation of treatment response and clinical development, readers are able to determine the effectiveness of pain management techniques and modify treatment plans as necessary to maximise therapeutic results.

Readers are advised to swiftly engage healthcare practitioners in the event of poor pain alleviation or unexpected bad effects. This will help to promote personalised interventions and avoid potential hazards connected with pain management measures. Furthermore, research into complementary and alternative medicine methods to pain management is something that should be taken into account in order to address the variety of clinical presentations and individual responses to different treatment interventions.

For the purpose of managing canker sore pain, it is necessary to have a thorough awareness of the various therapy modalities, clinical considerations, and the necessity of customised patient-centered methods that put safety and efficacy first. Through providing readers with useful tips and direction, the pain management techniques presented here hope to offer a thorough guide for reducing the burden of symptoms and creating an atmosphere that promotes quicker mucosal healing, so lessening the subsequent effects of canker sores on oral health and function.

The Role of Antibiotics in Treatment

Examining the possible function of antibiotics in treating these recurrent oral mucosal lesions is crucial as we dive into the comprehensive care of canker sores. When it comes to treating canker sores, antibiotics have generated a lot of discussion and attention. However, using antibiotics effectively requires careful consideration of their indications, potential advantages, and drawbacks. This chapter seeks to clarify the situations in which antibiotics may be administered for canker sores as well as their function in the larger treatment scheme. It covers clinical issues, practical applications, and common misconceptions.

The mainstay of contemporary medicine, antibiotics are pharmacological substances that work to prevent bacterial growth and reproduction in order to treat bacterial infections. Antibiotics are a viable intervention in the setting of canker sores to treat the infectious and inflammatory factors that may contribute to the aetiology and aggravation of these oral mucosal lesions.

Antibiotics are a broad class of pharmaceuticals used in the treatment of canker sores. They work by targeting bacterial pathogens and reducing the likelihood of exacerbating mucosal inflammation and infection. Through the targeting of particular bacterial cell components, they obstruct the growth and reproduction of these organisms, hence aiding in the resolution of underlying bacterial illnesses.

Antibiotic use for canker sores depends on whether or not secondary bacterial infections are present, as these can impede the healing process of these recurrent oral lesions. Although canker sores are generally thought to have a non-infectious genesis, those who have them may be more vulnerable to bacterial superinfection due to impaired oral mucosal integrity and the existence of predisposing variables such immunological dysregulation or oral trauma.

Antibiotics are used in these cases as a therapeutic adjuvant to treat the infectious factor and hasten the healing of the mucosa.

Antibiotic therapy's historical development has transformed the field of infectious disease management and ushered in a new era in the management of bacterial illnesses. An important turning point in the history of medicine was Alexander Fleming's 1928 discovery of penicillin, the first antibiotic. This discovery opened the door for the creation of a broad range of antibiotics with a variety of clinical uses and activity spectra.

When using antibiotics to treat canker sores, a thorough evaluation of the clinical setting is required. This evaluation should include the extent of oral lesions, the existence of concurrent systemic conditions, and any risk factors that may increase the likelihood of developing secondary bacterial infections. Moreover, the prudent use of antibiotics requires a customised strategy that takes into account the range of bacterial pathogens linked to oral infections as well as the patient's clinical response to particular antimicrobial drugs.

In clinical settings, the administration of antibiotics for canker sores is generally limited to instances where there is proof of secondary bacterial superinfection, as indicated by purulent exudates, systemic infection symptoms, or worsening mucosal inflammation that is not responding to standard non-antibiotic treatments. Antibiotics are used in the real world to treat canker sores, which highlights their supportive role in treating bacterial infections that could impede the clinical course of these oral lesions. This promotes faster mucosal healing and lessens the burden of symptoms.

One of the most common misconceptions regarding the use of antibiotics in the treatment of canker sores is that they should be prescribed without a strong clinical justification. Differentiating between the initial non-infectious cause of canker sores and the secondary bacterial infections that are superimposed on them is crucial since the appropriate use of antibiotics depends on the existence of clear clinical signs indicating bacterial involvement.

It is critical to emphasise the complex function that antibiotics play in treating the possible infectious elements that may be the cause of these recurrent oral mucosal lesions as we negotiate the landscape of canker sore care. The use of antibiotics requires a discriminating strategy that depends on a thorough evaluation of clinical signs that point to bacterial superinfection. This allows for the development of interventions that are specific to the patient's clinical situation and response to therapy.

The following chapters will further explore the complex field of canker sore treatment, including various treatment techniques, clinical considerations, and patient-centered strategies designed to promote mucosal healing and reduce the symptom burden associated with these recurrent oral lesions.

When to Consider Cauterization

Title:

:

Comprehending the cauterization procedure and its possible need is essential for the holistic treatment of canker sores. Cauterization is a therapeutic option that should be carefully considered, especially when non-invasive conventional treatments may not be sufficient to relieve the burden of symptoms associated with recurrent oral mucosal lesions. Examining the uses, advantages, and drawbacks of cauterization offers important insights into how it fits into the larger treatment plan, enabling medical professionals and those with canker sores to make well-informed decisions about how to treat them.

:

1. Cauterization
   2. Recurrent oral mucosal lesions
   3. Therapeutic intervention
   4. Indications
   5. Benefits
   6. Limitations

:

Cauterization:

In the context of managing canker sores, "cauterization" refers to the intentional application of heat, electricity, or chemical agents to the oral mucosal tissue that is affected, with the main goal being the induction of localised tissue damage. Through the initiation of a controlled inflammatory response and the facilitation of the building of a protective eschar, this method aims to enhance healing and potentially shorten the duration and severity of canker sore symptoms.

Recurrent Oral Mucosal Lesions:

Recurrent oral mucosal lesions are a group of inflammatory and ulcerative disorders that affect the oral cavity. They are distinguished by the emergence of painful, non-communicable ulcers and periodic flare-ups of oral mucosal inflammation. These lesions typically appear as one or more oral cavity ulcers that last for varying lengths of time and frequently reoccur, which adds to significant discomfort and functional impairment.

Therapeutic Intervention:

Therapeutic intervention refers to a wide range of medical and dental procedures that are intended to reduce the severity of symptoms and facilitate the resolution of underlying pathological conditions. These procedures may include behavioural, surgical, or pharmacological approaches that are customised to the patient's clinical circumstances and response to treatment.

Indications:

The terms "indications" in relation to cauterization refer to the clinical parameters and situations that justify the use of this therapeutic approach in the treatment of canker sores. These include the degree, duration, and refractoriness of oral lesions, as well as the patient's response to standard non-invasive therapies.

Benefits:

The advantages of cauterization centre on its ability to accelerate the healing process for canker sores by the induction of localised tissue death, the reduction of the symptomatic duration and severity of oral lesions, and the possible reduction of recurrence frequency. In addition, cauterization might encourage the development of a protective eschar, which would aid in mucosal healing and lessen pain related to canker sores.

Limitations:

The drawbacks of cauterization include the possibility of pain during the procedure, the possibility of unintentional tissue injury, and the requirement for exact administration and controlled tissue destruction. Furthermore, the clinical responsiveness of the patient, the nature of the oral lesions, and the existence of risk factors affecting the course of treatment can all affect how effective cauterization is.

Although cauterization is a medical and procedural process, it can be thought of as a controlled fire that makes room for renewal. The goal of cauterization is to start a regulated inflammatory response and tissue regeneration, similar to how controlled fires in forests remove overgrowth and promote new growth. This can speed up mucosal healing and maybe lessen the amount of symptoms associated with canker sores.

Conclusion:

A comprehensive understanding of cauterization's procedure, possible advantages, and clinical situations that call for its use offers a nuanced viewpoint on the treatment of canker sores. By providing information on the indications, advantages, and limitations of cauterization, medical professionals and patients with canker sores can make well-informed decisions about whether or not to incorporate this therapeutic approach into their treatment plans.

Immunosuppressants and Canker Sores

Aphthous ulcers, another name for canker sores, are a common oral mucosal ailment that affects the lining of the mouth and is characterised by painful, recurring ulcerations. Even though canker sores are benign, they can cause considerable discomfort and functional impairment, especially if they occur frequently or last for extended periods of time. Healthcare professionals and patients with chronic canker sores face a great deal of difficulty in managing this issue because traditional treatment approaches may not be sufficient in reducing the severity of symptoms and preventing recurrences. As a result, investigating alternate treatment approaches, including immunosuppressive medication, becomes essential for the holistic treatment of persistent canker sores.

The main problem with treating chronic canker sores is that traditional non-immunosuppressive therapy approaches are not very effective in providing long-term symptom alleviation or preventing recurrences. A paradigm shift in the treatment approach is required to address the underlying immunopathogenic mechanisms driving the recurrent nature of chronic canker sores because some patients still experience frequent and debilitating ulcerative episodes despite the availability of topical and systemic agents targeting inflammation, pain, and mucosal healing.

People who are plagued by chronic canker sores may experience ongoing discomfort, diminished oral function, and a lower quality of life if the problem of poor management is not addressed. The repeated nature of canker sores has emotional and psychological consequences, such as increased worry, social inhibition, and decreased self-esteem, in addition to physical discomfort. The financial burden of repeated medical visits, prescription costs, and lost productivity also exacerbates the effects of untreated chronic canker sores, highlighting the critical need for efficient long-term management techniques.

One potentially effective strategy for regulating the abnormal immune responses linked to the aetiology of chronic canker sores is the use of immunosuppressants. Immunosuppressants have the ability to produce a long-lasting remission, lessen the frequency of ulcerative episodes, and lessen the symptom burden that refractory canker sore sufferers endure by focusing on the dysregulated immune pathways that underlie mucosal inflammation and ulceration.

Immunosuppressant use in the treatment of chronic canker sores requires a thorough assessment of the patient's clinical profile, which includes the frequency and severity of ulcerative episodes, the patient's response to conventional treatment, and the existence of other medical disorders. Choosing the right drugs, dosage schedules, and monitoring procedures are all part of a customised strategy for immunosuppressant treatment that maximises effectiveness while lowering the risk of side effects and long-term issues.

Evidence-based support for the effectiveness of immunosuppressants in the treatment of chronic canker sores comes from observational studies and clinical trials that show a significant decrease in ulcerative frequency, severity, and healing time after starting immunosuppressant medication. Moreover, immunosuppressants' ability to treat the immunopathogenic cause of persistent canker sores is demonstrated by the prolonged remission they produce, providing a novel therapy option for patients with refractory illness.

Apart from immunosuppressants, biologic medicines that target distinct immune pathways linked to mucosal inflammation and ulceration are other treatment modalities that can be used as an adjuvant in the management of chronic canker sores. The development of personalised immunomodulatory methods and precision medicine may expand the range of available treatments even more, offering specialised care for patients whose immunopathogenic profiles differ and contribute to their canker sore burden.

To sum up, the use of immunosuppressants in the treatment of chronic canker sores represents a paradigm change in the way that the immunopathogenic causes of this illness are addressed. Using these medicines' immunomodulatory qualities, medical professionals can work to reduce the frequency of ulcerative episodes, achieve lasting remission, and lessen the burden of symptoms that people with refractory canker sores endure. When combined with continuing research efforts to clarify the immunologic cause of canker sores, the prudent use of immunosuppressants has the potential to completely alter the course of treatment and provide a glimmer of hope for individuals struggling with the management of chronic canker sores.

Diagnosis and Professional Care

Working With Your Dentist or Doctor

Canker sore management requires effective communication between patients and healthcare professionals. It is critical that both patients and healthcare professionals can clearly communicate their symptoms and concerns in order to provide appropriate diagnosis and treatment recommendations.

Many people find it difficult to explain their canker sore symptoms to their dentist or physician, which can result in miscommunication and less than ideal treatment results. Prolonged discomfort and delayed recovery may ensue from this.

Patients may not obtain the right care if they are unable to adequately express their symptoms and concerns, which could result in continued pain and discomfort. In addition to raising healthcare expenses and maybe adding to the patient's stress, misunderstandings can result in pointless tests or treatments.

Patients should be equipped with the information and abilities necessary to interact with their healthcare professionals in an efficient manner in order to resolve this problem. This may result in a more precise diagnosis, individualised treatment regimens, and better canker sore management all around.

There are various proactive measures that patients can take to improve their communication with their dentist or physician. First and foremost, it is crucial to record the frequency, length, and features of canker sores encountered in order to prepare for the appointment. The healthcare provider may get useful insights from this information. Patients should also be ready to talk about any possible causes or aggravating factors for their canker sores, such as dietary choices or dental hygiene routines. It's crucial for patients to get clarification as needed and look for further information if they have any doubts about the recommendations or course of treatment that their healthcare professional has given them.

Studies have indicated that patients' health results are enhanced when they participate actively in discussions with their healthcare providers. Patients who communicate their symptoms and concerns clearly have a greater chance of receiving individualised treatment programmes that cater to their individual needs, which can improve their quality of life and effectively control their symptoms. Moreover, people' thorough information sharing may be valued by medical professionals as it might lead to a quicker and more precise diagnosis.

While enabling individuals to connect with their healthcare providers efficiently is the main goal, it's as critical that healthcare providers are open to receiving concerns from patients. Healthcare professionals can guarantee that patients feel comfortable sharing their symptoms and needs for canker sore management by creating an environment that is open and collaborative.

In conclusion, good communication between patients and medical professionals is critical to the best possible treatment of canker sores. Patients can take charge of their care and help to enhance treatment outcomes by being prepared for appointments, participating actively in conversations, and asking questions when necessary. It is the responsibility of healthcare personnel to foster an atmosphere that promotes candid communication and teamwork, guaranteeing that patients feel appreciated and acknowledged in the treatment of their canker sores.

Understanding Medications and Prescriptions

Anyone looking for efficient management techniques must be aware of the drugs and prescriptions that are frequently used to treat canker sores. Patients are better able to understand the intended use, possible risks, and anticipated results of the drugs they are prescribed, which promotes informed decision-making and active engagement in their treatment regimens.

The following terms are crucial for comprehending the medications and prescriptions used in canker sore management:

1. Analgesics
2. Anti-inflammatory drugs
3. Antimicrobial agents
4. Topical corticosteroids
5. Oral rinses and mouthwashes

1. - Definition: Pain is a common symptom of canker sores, and analgesics are drugs made to relieve it.

- Detailed Explanation: These drugs function by obstructing the nervous system's ability to transmit pain signals, which in turn lessens the patient's sense of canker sore discomfort.

Relevance: By comprehending the function of analgesics, patients can better manage their canker sores and expect pain alleviation, which will enhance their quality of life overall as the sore heals.

2. - Definition: Anti-inflammatory medications are prescription medications that lessen inflammation, which is a crucial factor in the onset and spread of canker sores.

- Detailed Explanation: These drugs reduce the local inflammatory reaction linked to canker sores by blocking the action of inflammatory mediators such prostaglandins and leukotrienes.

Relevance: Patients can expect a decrease in pain, swelling, and redness by understanding how anti-inflammatory medications work, which can speed up recovery and enhance comfort.

3. - Definition: Antimicrobial agents are compounds that either stop or eliminate microorganisms, such as fungus and bacteria, which are frequently linked to the aggravation of canker sores.

- Detailed Explanation: By specifically targeting and interfering with bacteria' essential functions, these drugs stop them from proliferating and lower the chance of subsequent infections in canker sores.

Significance: Comprehending the function of antimicrobial agents enables patients to recognise the significance of upholding dental hygiene and adhering to recommended procedures in order to reduce the likelihood of recurrent infections, thereby facilitating efficient care of canker sores.

4. - Definition: Drugs called topical corticosteroids are injected straight into the damaged oral mucosa in order to reduce inflammation and encourage healing.

- Detailed Explanation: By inhibiting the local immune response, these drugs lessen the pain, edema, and inflammation brought on by canker sores while promoting tissue regeneration and healing.

Relevance: Patients who are knowledgeable with topical corticosteroids are better able to identify potential adverse effects as well as expected therapeutic effects, which promotes informed use and adherence to treatment plans.

5. - Definition: Often prescribed to maintain dental hygiene and relieve the symptoms of canker sores, mouthwashes and oral rinses are fluids that clean and soothe the oral cavity.

- Detailed Explanation: During bouts of canker sores, these solutions may contain antiseptic, analgesic, or anti-inflammatory drugs, which offer localised relief and support the health of the oral mucosa.

Relevance: By comprehending the function and ingredients of mouthwashes and oral rinses, patients can more successfully include these adjunctive therapies into their regular oral hygiene regimens, which helps to relieve symptoms and promote overall oral health.

Patients are able to comprehend the therapeutic meaning and practical application of canker sore treatments better when they make connections between them and topics they already know. As an illustration, using analgesics is similar to taking headache pain medications; both involve the goal of reducing discomfort. Antimicrobial drugs play a similar role to antibiotics in treating bacterial infections, underscoring the significance of following recommended treatment plans for optimal outcomes.

Comprehending the workings and intended effects of pharmaceuticals designed to treat canker sores encourages patient participation and adherence, which in turn improves quality of life and symptom management during canker sore episodes.

—-

I've included a thorough description of the actions and negative effects of some common drugs recommended for canker sores. Please let me know if you would want to see more sections or if there are particular subjects you would like to see more of.

When Surgery Is Considered

Phthous ulcers, another name for canker sores, are excruciating lesions that appear on the oral mucous membranes. Even though canker sores usually heal on their own in one to two weeks, some people may endure severe, recurrent, or abnormally big sores that have a major negative influence on their quality of life. In some situations, addressing these difficult symptoms with surgery might be a good alternative. This section will address situations where surgery may be required, describing the possible repercussions of treating these severe conditions without surgery and suggesting workable alternatives backed by data or expected results.

When it comes to canker sores, the biggest issue that requires surgery is when there are severe, recurrent lesions that seriously hinder a person's ability to chew, speak, and take care of their teeth. These lesions may cause chronic pain and suffering if they are very large, sluggish to heal, or resistant to standard therapies. Sometimes the placement of the canker sores—on the tongue or throat, for example—may present further difficulties, making the effect on the person's day-to-day functioning even worse.

Patients may continue to suffer from excruciating pain, have trouble eating and speaking, and have a limited capacity to maintain oral hygiene if these severe and recurring canker sores are not treated surgically. A lower overall quality of life, anxiety, and mental suffering might also result from these lesions' ongoing presence. The effects of treating these severe instances may also be worsened by the possibility of subsequent infections and longer healing times.

One practical option for treating severe and recurrent canker sores is surgery. These difficult manifestations can be successfully managed with procedures including laser therapy, corticosteroid injections, and surgical excision of the afflicted tissue, which relieve discomfort and hasten healing. Furthermore, the goal of surgical intervention is to stop these serious lesions from coming back, which will assist the affected people in the long run.

A thorough evaluation by a qualified oral and maxillofacial surgeon or oral medicine expert is required prior to the implementation of surgical intervention for the treatment of severe canker sores. To choose the best surgical strategy, a comprehensive assessment of the lesions and the patient's medical history is carried out prior to the treatment. The actual surgery is carried out carefully and precisely, frequently as an outpatient operation while the patient is under local anaesthesia to minimise discomfort.

The patient receives post-operative care and guidance for best healing after the surgical procedure. This could involve following strict dental hygiene guidelines, changing one's diet, and taking prescription drugs as directed. The healthcare professional schedules routine follow-up visits to assess the healing process and handle any issues or difficulties that may develop.

Surgical intervention has been shown to be effective in treating severe canker sores; multiple studies have reported significant pain alleviation, improved healing, and decreased recurrence risk after these treatments. Specifically, laser therapy has demonstrated encouraging results in the treatment of big and recalcitrant canker sores, facilitating a quicker healing process and improving patient comfort. Furthermore, it is impossible to overstate the psychological effects of surgically relieving patients of the burden of severe canker sores since they feel better emotionally and regain a sense of normalcy in their daily lives.

Although surgery is a useful option for treating severe and recurrent canker sores, other options might also be taken into account depending on the specifics of each case. These could be targeted immunomodulatory therapy, sophisticated pharmacological therapies, or adjuvant medications meant to address systemic aspects underlying the development of these difficult lesions. It is imperative to acknowledge, nevertheless, that in many instances, surgery is still the best course of action for bringing about permanent relief and managing severe canker sores over the long term.

To sum up, a crucial component of all-encompassing canker sore care is taking surgical intervention into account for severe canker sores. People can feel significantly less pain, have better oral function, and regain a sense of well-being by treating the underlying causes and lessening the effects of these difficult manifestations with precise and focused surgical operations. The incorporation of surgical intervention as a strategic element in the management of canker sores highlights the dedication to improving the general well-being of individuals impacted by these incapacitating oral diseases.

—-

This chapter has discussed the need for surgical intervention to treat severe and recurrent canker sores. It has also outlined the possible repercussions of treating these instances without surgery and offered workable treatments that are backed by data or expected results. A thorough grasp of surgery as a critical component of canker sore care enables patients and medical professionals to make well-informed choices and explore practical approaches to treating these difficult presentations.

The Role of Dental Hygiene

Aphthous ulcers, another name for canker sores, can be prevented and managed with careful dental hygiene. It is crucial to comprehend the relationship between dental hygiene habits and the development of canker sores since these excruciating lesions have the potential to greatly lower a person's quality of life.

It is asserted that managing and preventing canker sores can be achieved by practising good dental hygiene. People can improve their overall dental health and well-being by reducing the frequency and severity of these oral lesions by following recommended oral care procedures.

Canker sore development and poor dental hygiene have been shown to be related by research on a regular basis. Research have demonstrated that poor oral hygiene, such as insufficient brushing and flossing, can cause food particles and germs to build up in the oral cavity, which can facilitate the development of canker sores.

Because oral infections and germs have a part in both causing and aggravating canker sores, dental hygiene and these lesions are related. Bad dental hygiene fosters the growth of dangerous bacteria, which irritates and inflames the oral mucosa and puts people at risk for developing canker sores. Moreover, the accumulation of plaque and tartar may exacerbate tissue injury and weaken the body's defences against oral infections, making outbreaks of canker sores more likely.

Some may contend that canker sores can develop in people who maintain perfect oral hygiene, implying that causes other than oral hygiene may be involved in the development of these lesions. Furthermore, it has been determined that systemic diseases and genetic predisposition may also play a role in the formation of canker sores, suggesting that oral cleanliness may not be sufficient to prevent them entirely in all situations.

Although there is no doubt that genetic and systemic factors contribute to the susceptibility to canker sores, it is important to understand that keeping your teeth as clean as possible is still a critical part of reducing the likelihood and severity of these oral lesions. Implementing comprehensive dental care routines can help decrease the impact of canker sores and enhance oral health, even in persons with hereditary predispositions.

Research has also demonstrated the benefits of maintaining proper oral hygiene for the treatment of canker sores. Regular use of mouthwashes containing microorganisms and brushing and flossing have been linked to decreased inflammation and quicker healing of canker sores. In addition to treating the immediate symptoms of canker sores, good oral hygiene also promotes general oral health, which may have an impact on the frequency and severity of subsequent outbreaks.

In conclusion, it is impossible to overstate the importance of good dental hygiene in both managing and preventing canker sores. Even while systemic and hereditary factors may play a role in the formation of these oral lesions, practising good oral hygiene is still essential to reducing their frequency and fostering the best possible oral health. People can prevent canker sores and improve their general health by making oral hygiene a top priority.

Through the incorporation of dental hygiene principles into the therapy of canker sores, people are enabled to proactively mitigate the effects of these difficult oral manifestations and promote a healthy oral environment.

Insurance and Cost Considerations

Medical therapy of canker sores, sometimes referred to as aphthous ulcers, poses a complex challenge that goes beyond the mere discomfort that an individual may feel. Navigating the intricacies of insurance coverage and taking the related expenses of treatment into account are major components of this challenge. As such, it is critical for anyone seeking all-encompassing care and support to comprehend the significance of insurance and cost considerations in canker sore management.

The main concern here is the availability and cost of canker sore care, which includes diagnosis, treatment, and continuing care. Many people face barriers to receiving specialist care for canker sores because of insurance coverage constraints and the possible cost of different therapeutic methods. This difficulty frequently results in less-than-ideal canker sore care, which can worsen the physical and psychological effects on those who are afflicted.

The consequences of insufficient insurance coverage and financial obstacles in the treatment of canker sores are extensive. People can put off getting help from a professional, which could cause them to suffer longer and have a lower quality of life. In addition, the financial burden of paying for treatments out of pocket can lead to extra stress and anxiety, which can negatively affect the general wellbeing of those with canker sores. Financial difficulties might often prevent people from seeking the essential care, which could endanger their oral health and exacerbate canker sore breakouts.

A multimodal approach is required to address the issues with insurance coverage and economic considerations in the management of canker sores. This strategy entails pushing for full insurance coverage of canker sore diagnostics, treatments, and aftercare activities. Furthermore, encouraging financial assistance programmes and looking into cost-effective treatment options can improve access to care for those who are struggling financially.

Collaboration between insurance companies, regulatory agencies, and healthcare professionals is necessary to implement comprehensive insurance coverage for the management of canker sores. In order to guarantee that everyone has access to care, advocacy campaigns to broaden insurance coverage to include canker sore-related services—such as consultations with oral health specialists, diagnostic exams, and therapeutic interventions—are essential. Additionally, the financial burden of treatment expenditures for people with low incomes can be lessened by the creation of clear and patient-friendly financial support schemes.

Research and assessments of healthcare policies show that better financial support options and insurance coverage result in better canker sore results. For those with canker sores, increasing access to specialised care and treatments has been linked to better overall results, decreased disease burden, and improved treatment adherence. Furthermore, the execution of economical interventions and financial aid schemes may lessen the financial difficulties encountered by those pursuing all-encompassing management of canker sores.

It is crucial to take into account cooperative activities including healthcare facilities, advocacy organisations, and governmental agencies when looking into alternate options to address insurance and cost problems in canker sore management. In order to support people who require financial assistance for canker sore management, these initiatives may concentrate on negotiating favourable reimbursement rates for services related to canker sores, encouraging the development of reasonably priced generic medications, and facilitating partnerships with local resources.

In summary, managing insurance and financial concerns during the course of treating canker sores is essential to guaranteeing that those who are impacted have fair access to thorough care and assistance. The well-being of individuals affected by these difficult oral manifestations can be improved by advocating for increased insurance coverage, supporting cost-effective interventions, and creating patient-centered financial assistance programmes. These actions will help remove obstacles to accessing optimal management of canker sores.

Diet and Nutrition: The Canker Sore Connection

Foods to Avoid: Canker Sore Culprits

I: Introduction to the List

In order to effectively manage canker sores, it is essential to comprehend how dietary decisions affect the onset and severity of the problem. People can proactively modify their diets to reduce the incidence of canker sores by identifying particular items that have been shown to cause or exacerbate the condition. This list is an invaluable resource for understanding the complex connection between dietary components and the treatment of canker sores.

II: Presentation of the List

1. Citrus Fruits
2. Spicy Foods
3. Acidic and Pickled Foods
4. Nuts and Seeds
5. Chocolate
6. Coffee and Tea
7. Processed Snacks and Chips
8. Certain Dairy Products
9. Wheat-Based Products
10. Artificial Additives and Preservatives

III: Point Elaboration

a. Citrus Fruits

Citrus fruits are well known for being acidic, which can be especially hard on oral tissues, even though they are high in vitamin C and other healthy minerals. Citrus fruits' high acidity can irritate the mouth's fragile mucous membranes, which may result in the formation of canker sores. Frequent consumption of citrus fruits—like oranges, lemons, and grapefruits—can foster an environment where the development of canker sores is more likely, particularly in people who already have high oral sensitivity.

b. Spicy Foods

Eating meals high in capsaicin and other pungent substances, or spicy cuisine, has been associated with a higher risk of developing canker sores. These materials' abrasive properties have the ability to irritate and inflame the oral cavity, which may lead to the development of canker sores. In addition, the heat and spiciness of spicy meals can worsen already-existing canker sores, increasing discomfort and delaying healing.

c. Acidic and Pickled Foods

Pickles, vinegar-based sauces, and fermented goods are examples of acidic and pickled foods that have been linked to the exacerbation of canker sores. These foods' high acidity levels have the potential to dissolve the oral mucosa's protective layer, making it more susceptible to damage and the development of canker sores. In addition, pickles containing preservatives and flavourings may cause negative reactions in people who are prone to canker sores, making them more common.

d. Nuts and Seeds

Although seeds and nuts are known for their high nutritious content, several types may be problematic for those who are prone to canker sores. When chewed, the rough texture of nuts and seeds can cause tiny tears in the oral mucosa, which may lead to the formation of canker sores. Furthermore, the leftover particles from these foods may become trapped in oral fissures, acting as irritants to prolong the agony associated with canker sores and impede their healing.

e. Chocolate

Chocolate has ingredients linked to the worsening of canker sores, despite its allure as a decadent treat. Chocolate's high sugar level, theobromine concentration, and caffeine content can upset the delicate balance of dental health, causing inflammation and making canker sores more likely to occur. Moreover, some chocolate types' abrasiveness can mechanically harm oral tissues, making the treatment of canker sores even more difficult.

f. Coffee and Tea

Cattle and tea drinking, especially in large quantities, has been associated with a higher risk of canker sores. These drinks' acidic content, together with their tannin and caffeine content, can harm teeth and increase the risk of developing canker sores. Furthermore, these drinks' high temperatures have the potential to injure the oral mucosa thermally, aggravating canker sores already present and delaying their healing.

g. Processed Snacks and Chips

Many artificial flavours, preservatives, and additives found in processed snacks and chips can cause negative reactions in people who are prone to canker sores. These snacks' high salt level has the potential to dry oral tissues, leaving them more vulnerable to damage and the development of canker sores. Further complicating the care of canker sores is the abrasive texture of some snacks, which can cause mechanical stress to the sensitive oral mucosa.

h. Certain Dairy Products

Dairy products are a great way to get vital nutrients, but some types have been linked to making canker sores worse. Goods like yoghurt with a lot of sugar and aged cheeses can upset the oral flora, which can lead to the development of canker sores. Furthermore, several proteins found in dairy products have been related to immune system regulation, which may make sensitive people more susceptible to developing canker sores.

i. Wheat-Based Products

Products made from wheat, especially those that include gluten, have been linked to an increase in canker sores in those who have celiac disease or gluten sensitivity. Consuming gluten can worsen oral health by inducing an inflammatory response that makes canker sores more likely to occur. Moreover, the abrasive properties of some wheat-based products may mechanically damage the oral mucosa, aggravating the pain associated with canker sores.

j. Artificial Additives and Preservatives

Artificial additives and preservatives are widely found in processed foods, which has sparked worries about their possible effects on oral health, especially with reference to the incidence of canker sores. Some additives, such benzoates and sulfites, have been found to be vulnerable individuals' triggers for canker sores. The combination of these compounds and the inflammatory reaction they cause can lead to an environment that is favourable for the development and persistence of canker sores.

IV: Evidence and Testimonials

Numerous scientific studies and clinical observations show the link between dietary variables and the incidence of canker sores. Research has repeatedly shown how some foods can cause or exacerbate canker sores, providing insight into the complex relationship between dietary decisions and dental health. Moreover, first-hand reports from people who experience recurring canker sores highlight the significant effect that dietary changes have in easing symptoms and lowering the frequency of canker sore episodes.

V: Practical Applications

Equipped with a thorough comprehension of the dietary factors linked to the exacerbation of canker sores, people can utilise this knowledge to make well-informed dietary decisions that promote optimal oral health. Through deliberate avoidance or reduction of the listed foods, people can both prevent canker sores from occurring in the first place and lessen the discomfort that comes with already-existing sores. Moreover, including healthy and resilient oral substitutes in one's diet might encourage dental healing and resilience, giving people the confidence to actively treat their canker sores.

VI: Seamless Transitions

A comprehensive approach that includes both dietary adjustments and complete oral care practises is necessary due to the complex and dynamic interplay between dietary factors and the management of canker sores. After delving into the complex processes that lead to the formation of canker sores, the next chapters will clarify the critical roles that diet, dental hygiene, and lifestyle changes play in accomplishing all-encompassing management of canker sores. Through the utilisation of the information provided in this compilation, readers can initiate a revolutionary trip towards becoming proficient in managing canker sores and recovering dental health.

The therapeutic potential of oral-friendly foods and dietary treatments in creating a resilient oral environment that reduces the incidence of canker sores and encourages optimal oral health will be discussed in the upcoming chapter.

Healing Foods: What to Eat When You Have a Canker Sore

It is essential for those who want to reduce their canker sore symptoms and encourage healing to comprehend the role that nutrition plays in managing the condition. Through the identification of particular foods that facilitate the healing process, people can proactively maintain their oral health and reduce discomfort. This list functions as a thorough guide, providing information on the therapeutic qualities of different foods and their advantageous effect on the treatment of canker sores.

1. Aloe Vera
2. Honey
3. Coconut Oil
4. Yogurt
5. Leafy Green Vegetables
6. Oatmeal
7. Turmeric
8. Green Tea
9. Papaya
10. Blueberries

a. Honey

c. Respected for its antibacterial, anti-inflammatory, and wound-healing qualities, honey has been found to be an effective treatment for canker sores. Honey's healing properties are facilitated by the natural enzymes and antioxidants it contains, which also help to heal damaged tissue and lessen mouth ulcers. Applying unprocessed, raw honey to canker sores can reduce discomfort, stop infection, and hasten the healing process.

d. The effectiveness of honey in hastening the healing of mouth ulcers has been confirmed by scientific research, which attributes its advantages to its diverse biological properties. People who have used honey topically to treat canker sores have repeatedly attested to its calming properties, quick pain alleviation, and expedited healing periods.

e. People can manage canker sores naturally and holistically by incorporating raw, organic honey into their oral hygiene practises. It is a flexible and useful treatment for enhancing dental health and well-being due to its broad-spectrum healing abilities.

Continuing with the point elaboration:

b. Yogurt

c. Yogurt, which is high in probiotics and bioactive substances, is a great way to maintain dental health and lessen the discomfort associated with canker sores. Yogurt's probiotic bacteria, like Lactobacillus acidophilus, help maintain a healthy oral microbiome by inhibiting the growth of pathogenic bacteria and boosting immunity. Yogurt's soothing properties can also improve tissue healing, reduce irritation in the mouth, and hasten the healing of canker sores.

d. Studies have shown that yoghurt consumption is good for dental health, with its probiotic component contributing to better oral bacteria balance and fewer inflammatory reactions. People who have incorporated yoghurt into their diets have regularly reported less severe canker sores, faster healing rates, and general improvements in oral comfort.

e. Including probiotic-rich yoghurt in one's regular diet can offer a holistic, all-natural way of treating canker sores. It is a great ally in supporting oral wellness and promoting the healing of canker sores due to its soothing effects and good bacteria composition.

Continuing with the point elaboration:

b. Oatmeal

c. Rich in soluble fibre, vitamins, and minerals, oatmeal is a great aid in the treatment of canker sores and the advancement of oral healing. Oatmeal's calming, anti-inflammatory qualities can help with canker sore discomfort, soothe the mouth, and promote tissue healing. Oatmeal's high fibre content also promotes oral microbial balance and general oral health, which speeds up the healing of canker sores.

d. The positive impacts of oatmeal consumption on oral health have been highlighted by nutritional research, which highlights the food's ability to improve tissue repair, lower inflammation, and maintain a healthy balance of oral bacteria. People who have incorporated oats into their diets have regularly reported better oral comfort, faster healing, and a decrease in the severity of canker sores.

e. By incorporating oatmeal into one's everyday diet, one can manage canker sores naturally and holistically. It is an essential part of a diet that promotes dental wellness and the healing of canker sores because of its calming qualities and other health-promoting advantages.

Continuing with the point elaboration:

b. ** Preferred for its strong anti-inflammatory, antioxidant, and antibacterial qualities, turmeric provides helpful assistance in the treatment of canker sores and the advancement of oral healing. Curcumin, a bioactive substance present in turmeric,

Vitamins and Supplements for Prevention

The significance of vitamins and supplements in reducing the development and recurrence of these oral ulcers is a topic of significant interest in the pursuit of complete canker sore care. By being aware of the possible advantages of particular nutrients and dietary supplements in reducing the risk of canker sores, people can take proactive steps to maintain their dental health. The purpose of this chapter is to take a closer look at vitamins and supplements, investigating their potential for prevention as well as the scientific data supporting their effectiveness in treating canker sores.

The main claim that will be investigated is to the possibility that some vitamins and supplements can lessen the frequency and severity of canker sores, acting as preventative measures in advance.

The investigation of vitamins and supplements as a means of preventing canker sores starts with a consideration of vitamin B12, a crucial micronutrient that may have effects on dental health. Cobalamin, another name for vitamin B12, is an essential component of red blood cells, DNA synthesis, and neurological health. Due to its influence on immunological responses and role in maintaining the integrity of the oral mucosa, it may be relevant in preventing canker sores.

Research has indicated a possible correlation between a vitamin B12 deficiency and a higher vulnerability to mouth ulcers, such as canker sores. Because vitamin B12 supports the normal function of oral mucosal cells and plays a role in immunological modulation within the oral cavity, there is a complex interaction between vitamin B12 and oral health. Insufficient amounts of vitamin B12 can weaken the tissues in the mouth, making them more vulnerable to damage and the development of ulcers.

Moreover, because the pathophysiology of these oral ulcers has been linked to an imbalance in immunological responses, vitamin B12's immunomodulatory properties are very important for preventing canker sores. Canker sores may be less likely to occur in a balanced immunological milieu when vitamin B12 has the capacity to regulate immune activity, especially in the oral mucosa.

When analysing the claim regarding vitamin B12 and preventing canker sores, it is crucial to take into account counterarguments that contest the idea that a vitamin B12 shortage causes an increase in the frequency of oral ulcers. Although the possible effects of vitamin B12 deficiency on dental health have been recognised, a more thorough analysis of this micronutrient's specific function in canker sore prevention is warranted.

In response to counterarguments casting doubt on the direct correlation between vitamin B12 and the avoidance of canker sores, a comprehensive analysis of the complex nature of oral ulceration is necessary. Although a vitamin B12 deficiency may not be the only factor contributing to the development of canker sores, it is important to consider the impact on immune function and oral mucosal health. It is important to recognise the role that vitamin B12 plays in maintaining dental health in conjunction with other factors, rather than considering it as a stand-alone preventive treatment.

Extending the conversation about vitamins and supplements as a means of preventing canker sores, the emphasis now turns to the possible advantages of vitamin D in strengthening dental health and lowering the incidence of mouth ulcers. Fat-soluble secosteroid vitamin D is well known for its critical functions in immune system function, bone metabolism, and calcium homeostasis. Because of its immunomodulatory and anti-inflammatory qualities, which are essential to the resilience and health of the oral mucosa, it is relevant to the prevention of canker sores.

The immunomodulatory properties of vitamin D have been clarified by scientific studies, especially as they relate to dental health. The fact that vitamin D directly affects the immune responses in the oral cavity is demonstrated by the fact that oral mucosal cells have vitamin D receptors. Through its immune-modulating and anti-inflammatory properties, vitamin D helps to preserve the integrity of the oral mucosa and reduce inflammatory processes that can put people at risk for canker sores.

To sum up, the investigation into vitamins and supplements as a means of preventing canker sores highlights the complex relationship that exists between particular nutrients and dental health. Although vitamin B12 and vitamin D have been shown to have preventative qualities, it is important to understand that these nutrients' involvement in oral health are part of a complicated web of biological processes. Acknowledging the potential roles that these vitamins may have in immune modulation and oral mucosal integrity, people can take a comprehensive strategy to the prevention of canker sores that includes maintaining general oral health and eating habits.

People can proactively support their dental health and lessen the burden of canker sores by having a thorough awareness of the preventative potential of vitamins and supplements in the context of managing these mouth ulcers. To determine the exact mechanisms by which particular nutrients and dietary supplements affect the frequency and severity of canker sores, more research and clinical studies are necessary. This will open the door to more focused preventive measures and individualised methods of maintaining oral health.

The Role of Hydration in Canker Sore Management

This chapter's main goal is to clarify the critical role that hydration plays in the treatment of canker sores, highlighting the importance of hydration for both the development and healing of these oral ulcers. Through gaining a thorough grasp of how sufficient fluid intake affects the health of the oral mucosa, readers will be able to incorporate optimal hydration practises into their daily routines and help prevent canker sores.

In order to effectively manage canker sores, people must have a basic comprehension of the physiological mechanisms that underlie oral ulceration and the inextricable link between oral mucosal integrity and hydration. To make the most of the tactics discussed in this chapter, it is imperative to have the will to establish and maintain healthy drinking practises.

Effectively managing canker sores by maintaining optimal hydration requires a multimodal strategy that includes controlling fluid consumption, choosing hydrating drinks, and incorporating lifestyle choices that promote appropriate hydration. The main objective is to provide an internal environment that supports the health of the oral mucosa in order to reduce the risk of developing canker sores and to encourage the rapid healing of pre-existing ulcers.

1. The key to using hydration to manage canker sores is understanding the complex interactions between oral mucosal integrity and fluid balance. Maintaining the hydration condition of oral tissues is crucial for promoting their resilience and resistance to harm, including the development of canker sores. Because the inner lining of the mouth, or oral mucosa, is especially susceptible

to dehydration-induced damage, maintaining an appropriate fluid intake is essential for preventing canker sores.

The strategic monitoring of fluid intake is necessary for the proactive management of canker sores through hydration. People should make an effort to drink enough fluids each day to meet their demands for hydration, taking into consideration variables including age, gender, degree of physical activity, and ambient environmental conditions. Water, the main component of body fluids, is crucial for maintaining dental health since it is a vital part of saliva, which is essential for protecting and repairing the oral mucosa.

3. The body's defences against canker sores can be strengthened by choosing hydrated beverages that offer extra benefits to dental health in addition to water. Herbal beverages without added sugar, including licorice root tea or chamomile, provide calming and anti-inflammatory qualities that help ease dental pain and accelerate the healing of canker sores. Similarly, restoring essential nutrients and preserving oral mucosal hydration can be facilitated by coconut water, which is well-known for its electrolyte content and hydrating qualities.

4. Lifestyle choices that promote proper hydration, in addition to consuming fluids directly, are essential to the management of canker sores. Adding humidity to interior spaces can help prevent oral mucosal dehydration and lower the chance of developing canker sores, especially in dry or arid situations. Additionally, as both alcohol and caffeine have diuretic qualities that encourage fluid loss, limiting alcohol intake and moderation in caffeine intake can help maintain oral mucosal hydration over time.

- Tip 1: Keep a regular eye on your urine colour as a gauge of your level of hydration. Aim for pale yellow or straw-colored urine, as these indicate sufficient hydration.

- Tip 2: Eat foods that are high in water content, such oranges, cucumbers, and watermelon. These meals help to hydrate the oral mucosa and increase overall fluid consumption.

Be careful: Drinking too many sugary or acidic beverages can aggravate oral mucosal irritation and put people at risk of developing canker sores.

The assessment of oral mucosal health, which includes the reduction of canker sore frequency and severity as well as the rapid healing of pre-existing ulcers, can be used to evaluate the successful integration of hydration techniques for the management of canker sores. Furthermore, objective indicators of hydration status like urine specific gravity and osmolality can offer quantitative insights into how well fluid intake management is working.

When people have problems staying as hydrated as they should be in order to treat canker sores, one way to solve the problem is to identify any obstacles to being hydrated, like limited access to drinking water or underlying medical disorders that impact fluid balance. Hydration-related obstacles can be successfully resolved by working with healthcare providers to address these obstacles and customise hydration recommendations to meet individual needs.

In summary, the incorporation of water as a fundamental component of the management of canker sores highlights its critical function in maintaining the health of the oral mucosa and reducing the severity of these ulcers. Through the adoption of supportive lifestyle practises, the proactive regulation of fluid intake, and the choice of hydrating beverages, people can create an environment within themselves that supports oral health resilience and, in turn, empowers them to effectively and diligently manage canker sores.

Understanding Food Allergies and Sensitivities

Developing a comprehensive strategy for canker sore management requires an understanding of the relationship between dietary allergies and sensitivities and the development of canker sores. The incorporation of dietary concerns into techniques for managing canker sores recognises the possible impact of particular food ingredients on the health of the oral mucosa. Through explaining the complex relationship that exists between food allergies and sensitivities and canker sores, people can learn more about the specific triggers that may worsen or cause these mouth ulcers.

The main concern here is identifying and clarifying the role that dietary allergies and sensitivities play in the development of canker sores. People might not be aware of the possible link between the foods they eat and the development of canker sores, which could result in uncomfortable and frequent episodes of oral ulceration. It is difficult to manage canker sores proactively when people are unaware of particular dietary triggers, which feeds the loop of worsening symptoms and compromised oral mucosal health.

Ignoring the impact of food allergies and sensitivities on the onset of canker sores can lead to long-term oral pain, damaged oral mucosal tissue, and sluggish healing of pre-existing ulcers. Furthermore, the lack of specific dietary interventions may prolong the frequency and intensity of canker sore episodes, hence reducing the quality of life for those who have them. Moreover, prolonged exposure to triggers may exacerbate preexisting food allergies or sensitivities, which can have an effect on systemic health in addition to oral health.

The key to the answer is to outline a systematic procedure for determining and treating food allergies and sensitivities as possible causes of canker sores. Through the adoption of a customised nutritional evaluation and adjustment procedure, people can learn whether particular food items can be responsible for the development of canker sores. This method enables people to take proactive measures to reduce the negative effects of food triggers on oral mucosal health, which in turn creates an environment that promotes the prevention of canker sores and their faster healing.

There are various sequential processes involved in implementing individualised dietary adjustments to manage food allergies and sensitivities. First and foremost, people should do a thorough evaluation of their eating patterns and related incidence of canker sores, recording any possible associations between particular food consumption and the development of mouth ulcers. Then, with the help of medical professionals, implementing an elimination diet helps pinpoint particular dietary items that could act as canker sore triggers. Through this iterative approach, dietary triggers can be systematically identified and eliminated, opening the door to a customised eating plan that promotes the best possible oral mucosal health.

In terms of canker sore frequency, severity, and healing dynamics, the effective identification and management of dietary allergies and sensitivities as triggers for canker sores yields promising results. People who follow tailored trigger identification-based dietary changes frequently report fewer incidences of canker sores, less severe symptoms, and faster healing of pre-existing oral ulcers. In addition, putting into practise dietary plans customised for each person's dietary sensitivity promotes self-determination and proactive dental health maintenance, both of which enhance quality of life.

Although the suggested method places a strong emphasis on the individualised diagnosis and treatment of food allergies and sensitivities, other approaches include investigating more general dietary patterns and their possible effects on oral mucosal health. Adopting a comprehensive nutritional evaluation that takes into account variables including nutrient consumption, level of hydration, and overall nutritional balance could offer more information about reducing the risk of canker sores. Additionally, combining complementary therapy approaches—like probiotic supplementation and anti-inflammatory food ingredients—opens up new possibilities for enhancing oral mucosal resilience and reducing the effects of triggers.

Anti-inflammatory Diets and Canker Sores

Dietary therapies have drawn a lot of attention in the field of managing canker sores because of their ability to affect the frequency, severity, and healing dynamics of these oral ulcers. Of the wide range of dietary factors, anti-inflammatory diets have become a convincing approach to managing the susceptibility to canker sores. The focus on complete, unprocessed foods that are high in nutrients and bioactive substances with anti-inflammatory qualities is what defines an anti-inflammatory diet. This dietary strategy seeks to reduce systemic inflammation, which has an effect on the health of the oral mucosa and may therefore affect the development and treatment of canker sores.

The proposal that is being examined concerns the possible advantages of using an anti-inflammatory diet in decreasing the frequency and intensity of canker sores. This investigation aims to support the practicality of anti-inflammatory diets as a tactical element of all-encompassing canker sore care by clarifying the molecular mechanisms underlying inflammation in the context of oral ulceration and examining the effects of anti-inflammatory dietary patterns on oral mucosal health.

Essentially, the molecular mechanisms behind the formation of canker sores involve a complex interaction between tissue damage, inflammatory responses, and immunological dysregulation inside the oral mucosa. Under these circumstances, a thorough investigation of the impact of systemic inflammation on the development and progression of canker sores is necessary. Studies have outlined the function of pro-inflammatory mediators in the pathophysiology of oral ulcers, emphasising the possible significance of systemic inflammation in determining the intensity of symptoms and susceptibility to canker sores.

Systemic inflammation affects oral mucosal integrity in a complex way, since it is marked by an elevation of pro-inflammatory mediators and cytokines. The susceptibility of the oral mucosa to damage and ulceration can be increased due to immune homeostasis disruption and the exaggeration of inflammatory signalling pathways. Moreover, the coordination of inflammatory reactions in the oral mucosa could delay the healing of canker sores that are already present, worsening pain and compromising oral function.

On the other hand, it is critical to recognise the complex aetiology of canker sores and the possible drawbacks of linking systemic inflammation alone to oral ulcers. Although inflammation is unquestionably a crucial aspect of the pathophysiology of canker sores, a thorough knowledge of oral ulceration requires taking into account a variety of contributing factors, such as microbial impacts, genetic predispositions, and local trauma.

The recognition of the complex interactions among several etiological factors in the development of canker sores does not lessen the importance of systemic inflammation as a modifiable factor that may be targeted by dietary interventions. Instead, it emphasises the necessity of a multimodal strategy that incorporates many facets of the pathophysiology of canker sores, with a focus on comprehending the possible ameliorative benefits of anti-inflammatory foods in relation to oral ulceration.

Additional data from observational studies and clinical investigations supports the link between high-inflammatory-potential food patterns and increased mouth ulcer risk. On the other hand, strategies that support anti-inflammatory dietary patterns show potential for reducing inflammatory load and, consequently, for reducing the frequency and severity of canker sores.

As a result, research on anti-inflammatory diets as a tactical approach to managing canker sores highlights their ability to reduce systemic inflammation and improve the health of the oral mucosa. Through the alignment of dietary interventions with the objective of reducing pro-inflammatory processes, people can effectively utilise the therapeutic potential of anti-inflammatory diets to improve the overall management of mouth ulcers and reduce the susceptibility to canker sores. Thus, the incorporation of anti-inflammatory dietary approaches shows potential for developing a comprehensive guide for managing canker sores in their entirety, highlighting the critical role that dietary considerations play in the complex field of oral ulceration.

Meal Planning for Canker Sore Management

Meal planning for the management of canker sores is to create a dietary strategy that promotes oral mucosal health and reduces variables that increase the likelihood and intensity of canker sores. This book aims to offer a thorough blueprint for optimising dietary interventions in the context of canker sore care by creating meal plans and recipes that follow anti-inflammatory principles and meet the nutritional demands of those who are prone to canker sores.

Understanding the foundational ideas of an anti-inflammatory diet is necessary before beginning the process of meal planning for the treatment of canker sores. Furthermore, it's critical to have a complete awareness of the dietary variables that can affect the frequency and intensity of canker sores. Using the meal plans and recipes in this guide also requires having access to a wide variety of complete, unprocessed foods, as well as basic kitchen tools and supplies.

Meal planning for the management of canker sores involves carefully choosing and combining meals that have anti-inflammatory qualities, encourage the repair of oral mucosa, and address nutritional deficiencies that are frequently linked to the susceptibility to canker sores. This comprehensive review includes identifying important dietary components, developing balanced meal plans, and incorporating workable recipes that follow anti-inflammatory dietary guidelines.

1. Take into consideration any current dietary limitations or allergies while evaluating each person's unique eating habits and preferences. This stage lays the groundwork for customising meal plans to fit each person's requirements and tastes, which will improve adherence and satisfaction.

2. List and rank foods that have been shown to have anti-inflammatory effects, such as whole grains, fruits, vegetables, nuts, seeds, and fatty fish that is high in omega-3 fatty acids. These ingredients are the foundation for creating dishes and meal plans that reduce inflammation.

3. Verify that meal plans provide an adequate supply of protein, healthy fats, and complex carbs in addition to a macronutrient distribution that is balanced. Sustaining a balanced macronutrient composition is essential for maximising nutritional intake, promoting tissue healing, and preserving immune function.

4. Incorporate a variety of micronutrient-dense foods, such as leafy greens, citrus fruits, legumes, and berries, to help correct any possible nutritional deficiencies and promote the health of the oral mucosa. Zinc, folate, vitamin C, and vitamin E are micronutrients crucial for immune system regulation and tissue regeneration.

5. Put together a collection of recipes that follow anti-inflammatory dietary guidelines, emphasising the use of complete, unprocessed ingredients and cooking techniques that preserve the nutritional content of food. These recipes should be delectable, versatile, and practical for everyday meal preparation.

6. Implement the recommended food plans, taking into consideration individual tastes, lifestyle choices, and schedules. Meal plans should be sufficiently adaptable to allow for the alterations necessary to accommodate feedback and evolving dietary needs, since this will ensure sustained compliance and long-term nutritional achievement.

When meal planning, prioritise diversity and variation to provide a broad range of nutrients and bioactive substances that are essential for maintaining the health of the oral mucosa.

Stress the importance of maintaining proper hydration as a crucial component of canker sore treatment, and encourage consuming copious amounts of water and herbal teas.

- When introducing new foods or dishes, proceed with caution, particularly if you have any known allergies or dietary sensitivities. Consult a specialist if necessary. Steer clear of foods that are acidic or spicy since they may exacerbate the symptoms of a canker sore in individuals who are susceptible.

Evaluating overall oral mucosal health and general well-being, as well as monitoring the frequency and severity of canker sores, can corroborate the effectiveness of meal planning. Moreover, biochemical indicators of inflammation and nutritional status may serve as objective benchmarks for evaluating how well the meal programmes reduce systemic inflammation and strengthen immune function.

If there are challenges or barriers to adhering to the suggested meal plans, consider going back and examining the initial dietary habit and preference analysis to identify potential areas that could be adjusted. Additionally, get guidance from a qualified nutritionist to address any reoccurring issues and modify the meal planning approach as needed.

Holistic and Alternative Approaches

Herbal Remedies

I. Throughout history, people from many different nations and traditions have traditionally used herbal medicines to treat canker sores. A selection of herbal remedies that may be helpful for those with canker sores are included in the list below. Gaining knowledge of the underlying concepts and mechanisms of these treatments can help to improve their application and efficacy.

II. 1. Licorice Root
2. Chamomile
3. Aloe Vera
4. Sage
5. Echinacea

III.

a. Licorice Root

i. Licorice Root: An Overview

The Glycyrrhiza glabra plant yields licorice root, which has long been used in traditional medicine due to its antibacterial and anti-inflammatory qualities. Glycyrrhizin, the main ingredient, has strong anti-inflammatory properties that could help lessen the pain related to canker sores.

ii. The capacity of licorice root to impede the activity of pro-inflammatory enzymes is thought to be responsible for its anti-inflammatory qualities, which lessen the inflammatory response in the oral mucosa. Furthermore, by addressing underlying microbiological issues, licorice root has been researched for its ability to limit the growth of specific bacteria, which may help manage canker sores.

iii. Studies conducted in clinical settings have shown how effective licorice root is at lowering inflammation and accelerating the healing of wounds. Moreover, anecdotal information from people who have managed canker sores with licorice root preparations indicates a significant reduction in the sores' duration and suffering.

iv. Licorice root can be applied topically as a gel or as a mouthwash to specifically treat canker sores. Licorice root preparations can be incorporated into dental hygiene regimens as a useful and mild way to treat canker sores.

b. Rosemary

i. Chamomile: Taking Advantage of Its Healing Properties

Originating from the Matricaria chamomilla plant, chamomile is well-known for its analgesic and sedative qualities, which make it a popular option for treating disorders affecting the oral mucosa, such as canker sores.

ii. The anti-inflammatory and wound-healing properties of chamomile are attributed to its bioactive components, which include bisabolol and chamazulene. It has been demonstrated that these substances lessen inflammation and encourage tissue regeneration, which eases the pain brought on by canker sores.

iii. Studies have confirmed chamomile's anti-inflammatory and wound-healing qualities; results suggest chamomile may hasten the healing of mouth ulcers. Furthermore, people who have used topical treatments or oral rinses containing chamomile have reported less discomfort and faster healing of canker sores.

iv. People with canker sores can benefit from the medicinal properties of chamomile by using it topically as gels, mouth rinses, or teas. It is a promising herbal treatment for canker sore care due to its soothing nature and demonstrated effectiveness.

Aloe Vera: Revealing Its Restorative Properties c.

Aloe vera, which comes from the succulent plant Aloe barbadensis, has gained popularity as a herbal therapy for canker sore treatment because to its ability to heal wounds and reduce inflammation.

ii. The polysaccharides and bioactive compounds present in aloe vera gel contribute to its ability to accelerate wound healing and reduce inflammation. By modulating the inflammatory response and promoting tissue regeneration, aloe vera may offer relief from the pain and discomfort associated with canker sores.

iii. Studies investigating the therapeutic effects of aloe vera on oral ulcers have yielded promising results, highlighting its potential to expedite the healing process and alleviate symptoms. Testimonials from individuals who have used aloe vera-based products for canker sore management underscore its efficacy in providing relief and promoting oral mucosal health.

iv. Aloe vera gel can be applied topically to canker sores to harness its healing properties. Additionally, aloe vera-based mouth rinses may offer a practical and gentle approach to managing canker sores, providing individuals with a natural alternative for alleviating oral discomfort.

d. Sage

i. Sage: Tapping into Its Therapeutic Potency

Sage, derived from the Salvia officinalis plant, is revered for its antimicrobial and anti-inflammatory properties, making it a compelling herbal remedy for addressing canker sores.

ii. The bioactive compounds present in sage, such as rosmarinic acid and essential oils, exhibit potent antimicrobial and anti-inflammatory effects. These properties enable sage to combat microbial overgrowth and reduce inflammation within the oral mucosa, potentially contributing to the management of canker sores.

iii. Research studies have elucidated the antimicrobial and anti-inflammatory attributes of sage, highlighting its potential for mitigating microbial factors and alleviating inflammation associated with canker sores. Furthermore, individuals who have incorporated sage-based oral preparations have reported reduced pain and accelerated healing of canker sores.

iv. Sage can be harnessed in the form of mouth rinses or topical applications to target canker sores directly. Its dual action against microbial overgrowth and inflammation positions sage as a valuable herbal remedy for promoting oral health and managing canker sores.

e. Echinacea

i. Echinacea: Unveiling Its Immunomodulatory Effects

Echinacea, derived from the Echinacea purpurea plant, is renowned for its immunomodulatory properties, which have implications for managing conditions characterized by immune dysregulation, including canker sores.

ii. The bioactive compounds present in echinacea, such as alkamides and polysaccharides, exert immunomodulatory effects by modulating immune cell activity and cytokine production. By regulating immune responses, echinacea may help rebalance immune function within the oral mucosa, potentially influencing the development and resolution of canker sores.

iii. Research studies have substantiated the immunomodulatory effects of echinacea, suggesting its potential for modulating immune responses within the oral mucosa. Individuals who have integrated echinacea preparations into their canker sore management routines have reported reduced frequency and severity of outbreaks, indicating its influence on immune-mediated aspects of canker sore development.

iv. chinacea can be incorporated into oral preparations, such as mouth rinses or lozenges, to harness its immunomodulatory effects and potentially influence the immune dysregulation associated with canker sores. Its role in rebalancing immune function presents a distinctive approach to canker sore management, offering individuals an avenue to address underlying immune imbalances.

IV. As we delve into the intricate realm of herbal remedies, the multifaceted properties and therapeutic potentials of licorice root, chamomile, aloe vera, sage, and echinacea come to light, presenting a diverse array of options for canker sore management. Each herbal remedy offers unique mechanisms of action and practical applications, underscoring the rich tapestry of natural interventions available to individuals seeking comprehensive approaches to canker sore management. In the subsequent chapters, we will continue to explore the dynamic landscape of natural remedies, delving deeper into their potential benefits and practical implications for canker sore sufferers.

Acupuncture and Acupressure

I. Acupuncture and acupuncture have become well-known therapeutic modalities in complementary and alternative medicine that have the ability to reduce pain, encourage healing, and help the body regain its equilibrium. These age-old methods, which have their roots in traditional Chinese medicine, use qi, or vital energy, and the concepts of meridian theory to affect the body's energetic and physiological functions. Acupressure applies pressure on these acupoints to induce therapeutic effects, whereas acupuncture inserts tiny needles at predetermined acupoints. A thorough investigation is necessary to clarify the processes and practical consequences of the use of acupuncture and acupressure in the management of pain and promotion of healing, including the possibility of their effectiveness in treating canker sores.

II. Acupuncture and acupressure are effective methods of promoting healing and controlling pain, and they may provide alleviation from the agony that comes with canker sores.

III. A. Acupuncture: Revealing Its Healing Principles

i. Acupuncture's Mechanism: Modulating Pain and Balancing Qi Perception

The idea of qi, the life force that moves through the body's meridians, or energy corridors, is fundamental to the practise of acupuncture. Pain and sickness can be signs of imbalances or disturbances in the movement of qi, according to traditional Chinese medicine. Acupuncture seeks to stimulate particular meridians' acupoints in order to restore the balanced flow of qi, thereby addressing the underlying cause of pain and promoting healing.

ii. Acupuncture's Neurophysiological Impact: Adjusting Pain Signaling Pathways

The neurophysiological principles behind acupuncture's analgesic benefits have been clarified by recent study. Research has indicated that the stimulation of acupuncture triggers the release of endogenous opioids, including endorphins and enkephalins, which function as endogenous analgesics. Furthermore, acupuncture has been demonstrated to regulate pain signalling pathways within the central nervous system by modifying the activity of neurotransmitters and neurohormones involved in pain perception.

B. Acupressure: Using Meridian Stimulation to Its Full Potential

i. Meridian Theory and Acupressure: Impacting Physiological Function and Energetic Flow

Similar to acupuncture, acupressure is based on meridian theory and seeks to balance the body by influencing qi flow. Acupressure activates the meridians by applying pressure to particular acupoints, which helps the body's natural healing processes and allows qi to flow more freely.

ii. Acupressure's Physiological Effects: Managing Pain and Promoting Healing

Studies on acupressure's physiological effects have shown that it can influence how pain is perceived and facilitate the healing process. It has been discovered that acupressure causes the release of neurotransmitters linked to relaxation and pain alleviation, such as serotonin and endorphins. Acupressure has also demonstrated promise in lowering tense muscles, increasing blood flow, and strengthening the body's capacity for tissue regeneration and healing.

IV. A. Acupuncture: Clinical Research and Meta-Analytic Perspectives

i. Acupuncture's Clinical Effectiveness in Pain Management

Clinical studies examining the effectiveness of acupuncture in pain relief have shown that it is beneficial in reducing both acute and chronic pain. Acupuncture has been shown to be significantly more effective at relieving pain than sham acupuncture and standard care, according to meta-analyses of trials, underscoring its potential as a useful therapeutic tool.

ii. Treating Canker Sore Pain with Acupuncture for Oral Health

The analgesic and anti-inflammatory properties of acupuncture make it worth considering for its possible application in disorders affecting the oral mucosa, even though there hasn't been much research especially on the treatment of canker sores. The pain associated with canker sores may be lessened by acupuncture's capacity to alter pain perception and reduce inflammation, acting as an adjuvant to traditional treatments.

B. Acupressure: Clinical Uses and Empirical Support

i. Acupressure's Empirical Basis for Pain Relief

Research examining the effectiveness of acupressure in treating a range of ailments, including headaches, menstrual pain, and musculoskeletal discomfort, provides empirical support for the treatment's wide application as a non-invasive method. These research' encouraging results lend credence to acupressure's potential for pain and discomfort management.

ii. Examining Acupressure for Oral Ulcers: Consequences for the Treatment of Canker Sores

Although there isn't much study specifically on using acupressure to treat canker sores, the concepts of meridian stimulation and pain regulation that are part of acupressure point to its possible application in treating oral ulcers. Acupuncture's capacity to affect how people perceive pain and encourage relaxation may help those who have canker sores feel less uncomfortable and support their healing processes.

V.

A. Critiques of Acupuncture: Challenges and Skepticism

i. Methodological Limitations and Placebo Effects

The methodological rigour of acupuncture research has drawn criticism from some quarters, who point to difficulties in creating suitable control conditions and blinding techniques. Furthermore, there has been discussion on the contribution of placebo effects to acupuncture outcomes. Some have questioned the specificity of acupuncture's effects, questioning if they extend beyond placebo responses.

B. Acupressure: Issues to Take Into Account and Debates

i. Selected Empirical Studies in Particular Situations

A challenge in establishing the direct effectiveness of acupressure for oral mucosal disorders, such as canker sores, is the dearth of empirical data on the subject. Although acupressure has shown promise in treating a variety of pain disorders, its possible application for treating mouth ulcers should be interpreted cautiously due to the lack of focused studies in this area.

Section VI. A: Handling Methodological Issues Developments in the Study of Acupuncture

The scientific rigour of acupuncture studies has been improved by advances in study procedures, such as the use of strong placebo controls and creative neuroimaging approaches. The incorporation of neuroimaging techniques, such as functional magnetic resonance imaging (fMRI), has yielded vital clarification on the unique physiological actions of acupuncture and provided insights into the neurobiological mechanisms underlying its effects.

B. Setting Acupressure in Perspective: Applying Overall Effectiveness to the Treatment of Oral Ulcers

The general effectiveness of acupressure in pain reduction and relaxation calls for investigation in the context of managing oral ulcers, even though the lack of particular studies on the use of acupressure for canker sores calls for caution. Canker sore sufferers may find relief from their agony and faster healing from the modulatory effects of acupressure on pain perception and physiological systems.

VII. There is strong evidence to support the promise of acupuncture and acupressure as therapeutic treatments for pain management and healing as we explore their complex environment. The neurophysiological mechanics of acupuncture and the principles of meridian stimulation in acupressure provide complex insights into how they might be applied to address the complex nature of pain, including the discomfort that comes with canker sores. Although there have been criticisms and considerations, the growing body of empirical evidence and the development of research methodologies support the idea that acupuncture and acupressure are useful additions to the overall pain and healing processes, which may have consequences for people who are struggling to manage canker sores.

Aromatherapy and Essential Oils

In the field of holistic health and wellbeing, the use of essential oils and aromatherapy as supplementary and alternative therapies has attracted a lot of interest. Aromatherapy and essential oils have become well-known as promising modalities for symptom relief and general well-being because of their extensive historical background and wide range of therapeutic applications. A thorough analysis of the processes and practical consequences of aromatherapy and essential oils in managing canker sores is necessary to fully understand their potential in relieving discomfort and fostering oral mucosal repair.

Combining aromatherapy with essential oil application offers prospective ways to enhance oral mucosal healing and manage symptoms of canker sores, indicating their ability to provide relief from the pain associated with these oral ulcers.

A. Aromatherapy: Unveiling Its Therapeutic Mechanisms

i. Olfactory Stimulation and Neurophysiological Effects

The induction of olfactory stimulation by the inhalation of aromatic molecules obtained from essential oils is a fundamental aspect of aromatherapy treatment. The limbic system and the hypothalamus, which are areas linked to emotions, memory, and autonomic processes, are connected to the olfactory system, and these linkages highlight the potential for aromatherapy to affect both psychological and physiological processes. It has been demonstrated that inhaling particular essential oils can cause different neurophysiological reactions, such as relaxation, stress reduction, and mood modulation. These effects may help to lessen the mental and emotional discomfort that frequently accompanies the discomfort of a canker sore.

ii. Anti-inflammatory and Antimicrobial Properties of Essential Oils

A multitude of essential oils exhibit strong anti-inflammatory and antibacterial characteristics, which are pertinent in managing the inflammatory aspect of canker sores and reducing the likelihood of subsequent infections. Essential oils contain compounds called terpenes, phenols, and aldehydes that have anti-inflammatory properties. These compounds work by regulating the production of cytokines and blocking inflammatory mediators, which may lessen the discomfort and swelling that come with canker sores. Additionally, some essential oils' antibacterial properties may help stop or manage microbial colonisation in the oral cavity, promoting the healing of canker sores.

B. Essential Oils: Exploring Their Therapeutic Potential

i. Topical Applications of Essential Oils for Oral Mucosal Health

Applying essential oils locally to the oral mucosa offers a direct way to use their healing qualities to treat the symptoms of canker sores. Tea tree, chamomile, and lavender oils are examples of essential oils that have analgesic and anti-inflammatory qualities. These oils can provide specific relief from the pain and discomfort caused by canker sores while also acting as an anti-inflammatory to aid in the healing process of oral ulcers. The significance of essential oils for maintaining the health of the oral mucosa is further supported by their capacity to stimulate tissue regeneration and strengthen the local immune response.

ii. Psychological Impact and Stress Reduction

Because of the psychological effects of canker sores, which include discomfort, irritation, and poor oral function, symptom management must be approached holistically. Essential oils with anxiolytic and mood-enhancing qualities, including frankincense, ylang-ylang, and bergamot, may help lessen the emotional strain that comes along with the discomfort of a canker sore. These essential oils may support the body's natural healing processes and enhance the overall treatment of canker sore symptoms by promoting relaxation, lowering tension, and enhancing emotional well-being.

A. Efficacy of Aromatherapy in Pain Management and Healing

i. Clinical Studies on Aromatherapy for Pain Relief

Studies investigating the effectiveness of aromatherapy as a pain management tool have shown that it can reduce pain associated with a range of illnesses, such as neuropathic pain, postoperative pain, and musculoskeletal pain. Aromatherapy's ability to reduce pain has been linked to its ability to promote relaxation and modulate pain perception, underscoring its applicability in treating pain's complex nature, which includes the agony that comes with canker sores.

ii. Wound Healing and Tissue Regeneration

Research on the ability of essential oils to treat wounds has shown that they can speed up tissue restoration, lessen inflammation, and improve the healing process as a whole. Essential oils with potential to promote epithelialization and shorten wound healing times include lavender, geranium, and helichrysum oils. These discoveries may help resolve canker sores and lessen their negative effects on oral function.

B. Safety Considerations and Application Methods

i. Dilution and Safe Application of Essential Oils

Because essential oils are concentrated, they should be handled carefully and diluted appropriately if applied to the oral mucosa. Safe topical administration is ensured and the danger of negative reactions is reduced by diluting essential oils in carrier oils or water-based preparations. Respecting the suggested dilution ratios and application techniques is crucial to avoid irritation or sensitization, especially in the delicate oral mucosa.

ii. Individual Variability and Sensitivity

The importance of tailored techniques in aromatherapy applications is highlighted by the individual heterogeneity in response to aromatic compounds and essential oils. In order to ensure safe and efficient consumption, factors including allergies, sensitivities, and medical problems may affect a person's tolerance and response to particular essential oils. As such, careful evaluation and probable contact with healthcare professionals may be necessary.

A. Limited Standardization and Variability in Essential Oil Composition

It is difficult to evaluate the consistent therapeutic benefits of essential oils due to the absence of defined restrictions and compositional diversity. The effectiveness and safety of essential oils produced from various sources may be impacted by differences in their chemical profiles, which calls for caution when interpreting their use in clinical settings, including the treatment of canker sores.

B. Psychological Placebo Effects and Subjective Responses

Concerns about the possible impact of subjective reactions and psychological placebo effects on aromatherapy interventions have been voiced by critics. Individual reactions may vary due to the subjective nature of olfactory perception and the psychosomatic aspects of aromatherapy experiences. Therefore, it is important to critically evaluate the interpretability and repeatability of study findings in aromatherapy.

A. Quality Control and Authentication of Essential Oils

The authentication and standardisation of essential oils have been improved by developments in analytical methods and quality control procedures. The identification and measurement of important chemical components in essential oils is made possible by techniques like gas chromatography-mass spectrometry (GC-MS) analysis, which helps to guarantee the oils' authenticity, purity, and consistency between batches. These developments strengthen the dependability of essential oil uses in clinical and therapeutic settings by addressing issues with variability and quality assurance.

B. Integrating Subjective Experiences with Objective Measures

Although subjective sensations may have some influence in aromatherapy, combining qualitative evaluations with objective measurements provides a thorough method of assessing its therapeutic effects. A more nuanced understanding of the holistic effects of aromatherapy is made possible by combining self-reported outcomes with physiological and psychological parameters. This approach offers important insights into the potential relevance of aromatherapy in managing the symptoms of canker sores and promoting oral mucosal healing.

There is strong evidence to support the promise of aromatherapy and essential oils as therapeutic techniques for controlling the symptoms of canker sores and promoting oral mucosal healing as we explore their complex realm. Aromatherapy's neurophysiological effects and the many therapeutic benefits of essential oils provide complicated insights into how best to handle the intricacies of canker sore discomfort. Although there have been criticisms and concerns raised, the growing body of evidence, safety concerns, and improvements in quality assurance support the idea that aromatherapy and essential oils might be useful additions to the overall treatment of canker sore pain and oral mucosal health.

To summarise, the investigation of aromatherapy and essential oils as possible modalities for managing canker sores offers a thorough understanding of their therapeutic workings, clinical applications, and safety factors. Their wide range of characteristics, which include psychological impacts, the ability to heal wounds, neurophysiological effects, and anti-inflammatory actions, highlight their importance in addressing the complex nature of canker sore discomfort and promoting oral mucosal healing. The combination of aromatherapy and essential oils presents potential opportunities to improve the all-encompassing treatment of canker sores as the field of holistic healthcare develops, representing a holistic approach to fostering oral health and general well-being.

Homeopathy and Canker Sores

An alternative medical technique called homoeopathy provides a special method of treating a number of illnesses, including canker sores. Homeopathy gives exciting options for treating canker sore symptoms and encouraging oral mucosal healing because of its premise of "like heals like" and use of highly diluted natural medicines. This section will explore the fundamentals and uses of homoeopathy in the treatment of canker sores, looking at its therapeutic mechanisms and possible ramifications for people looking for all-encompassing approaches to oral health.

Because of their personalised and all-encompassing approach, homoeopathic remedies have the potential to address the underlying imbalances causing these oral ulcers and improve general health. They have shown promise in managing the symptoms of canker sores and promoting oral mucosal healing.

A. Homeopathic Principles and Individualized Treatment

i. Law of Similars and the Selection of Remedies

The foundation of homoeopathy is the idea of "like heals like," which is finding a homeopathic remedy that would cause symptoms in a healthy person that are similar to those the patient is experiencing. Homeopathic practitioners customise treatment regimens for canker sores based on the unique characteristics of the ulcers, including their location, appearance, and concomitant symptoms. By addressing the underlying constitutional and systemic imbalances that contribute to the development of canker sores, this method offers a customised and all-encompassing approach to managing symptoms.

ii. Potentization and Dilution of Remedies

Potentization, which includes vigorous shaking and successive dilution, is an essential step in the manufacture of homoeopathic remedies. With the goal of maximising the substances' energetic qualities while reducing their material concentration, this method yields very diluted medications that are thought to function on the body's delicate energy levels. The foundation of homeopathy's use of highly diluted remedies is the idea that the potentiation of the original substance through succussion can create a dynamic imprint that can elicit profound healing responses. This approach is in line with the holistic approach to treating the underlying causes of health conditions, such as canker sores.

B. Homeopathic Remedies for Canker Sore Management

i. Arnica montana: Addressing Trauma and Inflammation

One well-known homoeopathic treatment for disorders including trauma, bruising, and inflammatory responses is arnica montana. Arnica montana may be advised for people who have oral trauma, such as bites or injuries that occur unintentionally, in addition to the development of canker sores. Arnica montana's traditional usage in treating oral and mucosal disorders is supported by its potential to reduce the inflammatory processes linked to canker sores and facilitate tissue recovery.

ii. Borax: Managing Recurrent Canker Sores

Borax, a homoeopathic medicine made from sodium borate, is frequently taken into consideration for people who frequently get canker sores, particularly those who have heightened sensitivity to acidic or spicy foods. Borax use is characterised by symptoms such as recurrent mouth ulcers, increased irritation, and discomfort that is aggravated by specific food triggers. In homoeopathic practise, Borax is chosen on an individual basis because of its ability to address the underlying susceptibility and triggers that lead to recurrent canker sores.

A. Clinical Observations and Provings

i. Individual Responses and Provings of Homeopathic Remedies

In homoeopathy, provings are made by giving highly diluted medicines to healthy people in order to elicit and record their symptom profile. These demonstrations offer important new information on the typical symptoms and possible medical uses of homoeopathic treatments. Clinical observations and provings are important in developing a more nuanced understanding of the symptom patterns and individual responses related to canker sores. This understanding aids in the selection of homoeopathic remedies that are specifically designed to address the unique manifestations of oral ulcers.

    ii. Individualized Case Studies and Long-Term Management

Homeopathy places a strong emphasis on evaluating patients as a whole, taking into account all of their mental, emotional, and physical characteristics, in order to provide tailored case management. Long-term case studies and clinical observations of people treated with homoeopathy for recurrent canker sores provide insights into the possibility of long-term recovery, decreased frequency of outbreaks, and improved general health. Homeopathy's personalised approach highlights its applicability in managing the complex aspects of canker sores and promoting the long-term health of the oral mucosa.

    B. Safety Considerations and Practitioner Expertise

    i. Safety Profile of Highly Diluted Remedies

Homeopathic treatments have a good safety profile because of their large dilutions, which reduce the possibility of side effects from material concentrations. This safety consideration relates to the possibility of safely exploring homoeopathic options for managing canker sore symptoms without significant concerns regarding toxicity or interactions with conventional medications for individuals, including those with heightened sensitivity or underlying health conditions.

    ii. Professional Guidance and Individualized Consultations

Because homoeopathy is a personalised kind of treatment, it is crucial to seek advice from licenced professionals with homoeopathic experience. The ability of practitioners to perform thorough assessments, which include in-depth case-taking and constitutional evaluations, allows for the customised selection of homoeopathic remedies that are in line with each patient's unique symptom profile. This helps to provide efficient and individualised care for canker sores.

A. Skepticism and Limited Scientific Consensus

The limited scientific consensus and difficulties in determining the reproducibility of results in homoeopathic research have been brought up by homoeopathic critics. The integration of homoeopathic techniques into conventional healthcare paradigms, particularly the therapy of oral health disorders like canker sores, is hindered by the scepticism surrounding the mechanisms of action of homoeopathy and the interpretation of its clinical outcomes.

B. Placebo Effects and Contextual Influences

There has been discussion on the possible impact of contextual circumstances and placebo effects on how each person responds to homoeopathic treatment. Some who question the particular therapeutic effects of homoeopathic medicines beyond placebo responses contend that perceived improvements may be influenced by the subjective nature of symptom reporting and the impact of patient-practitioner relations.

A. Holistic Framework and Energetic Paradigm

Homeopathy's holistic approach to treatment, which takes into account the interdependence of the mental, emotional, and physical facets of health, provides a unique viewpoint on treating ailments like canker sores. The energetic paradigm that underpins homoeopathy highlights the complex interplay between the dynamic qualities of very diluted medicines and the individual's vital energy, which adds to the personalised and all-encompassing approach to oral mucosal health.

B. Patient-Practitioner Relationship and Therapeutic Alliance

In homoeopathy, the patient-provider connection highlights the significance of building a therapeutic alliance based on empathy, active listening, and cooperative decision-making. This method seeks to address each person's particular experiences and health issues while creating a welcoming environment for investigating homoeopathic remedies for the treatment of canker sores. The relationship between a patient and a practitioner goes beyond the prescription of medications; it also includes comprehensive assistance and direction specific to the patient's health.

The concepts of customised care, comprehensive evaluation, and the careful choice of highly diluted remedies become evident as we explore homoeopathy and its possible uses in the treatment of canker sores. These strategies are essential for addressing the complex issues surrounding oral mucosal health. Homeopathy's customised approach, based on the ideas of potentization and "like heals like," offers encouraging options for treating canker sore symptoms and promoting long-term dental health. Homeopathy's validity as a valuable component in the comprehensive management of canker sores is reinforced by its safety considerations, individualised consultations, and holistic framework, all of which acknowledge critiques and the need for ongoing research. This approach reflects a holistic approach to promoting oral health and overall well-being.

In conclusion, the investigation of homoeopathic treatments for the treatment of canker sores offers a thorough understanding of the tenets, uses, and safety concerns of homoeopathy in addressing the intricacies of oral mucosal health. Homeopathic remedies can be individually selected based on a patient's unique symptom profile and holistic assessment. This approach offers potential solutions for treating the symptoms of canker sores, maintaining long-term dental health, and boosting general well-being.

Stress Management Techniques

Stress frequently surfaces as a major trigger in the holistic management of canker sores, aggravating the frequency and severity of these oral ulcers. In order to give people practical tools for reducing stress-related canker sore aggravation, this section presents a variety of stress management practises. These methods seek to develop resilience, enhance emotional health, and lessen the influence of stress on the development and duration of canker sores by addressing the relationship between stress and dental health.

The stress management techniques presented herein encompass a diverse array of evidence-based approaches, each offering distinct pathways for individuals to navigate and alleviate stress in their lives. From mindfulness practices to cognitive-behavioral strategies, the following list provides a comprehensive overview of techniques tailored to the complex interrelationship between stress and canker sore management:

a. Mindfulness meditation is a powerful technique for reducing stress and its negative effects on dental health. It is based on the development of present-moment awareness and nonjudgmental observation. People who practise mindfulness can become more self-aware, reduce ruminating, and cultivate a sense of calmness in the face of everyday obstacles.

b. A practical method of reducing both physical and mental stress is progressive muscle relaxation, which is the methodical tensing and relaxing of muscle groups. People can lessen the physiological effects of stress by learning to identify and release muscle tension, which may limit the impact of stress on the development and aggravation of canker sores.

c. A fundamental element of cognitive-behavioral therapies, cognitive restructuring enables people to recognise and confront unhelpful thought patterns that lead to stress. People can control their emotional reactions and lessen the negative effects of stress on their dental health by rephrasing their stressful ideas and beliefs. This may break the cycle of stress-induced canker sore exacerbation.

d. Regular exercise, which includes both resistance and aerobic training, is a comprehensive strategy for reducing stress. Exercise's physiological and psychological effects, such as the production of endorphins and the development of stress resilience, might lessen the negative effects of stress on the frequency and intensity of canker sores and enhance general wellbeing.

a. Building emotional fortitude and social support systems provides a hedge against the damaging effects of stress on dental health. People can manage stress more skillfully and possibly lessen its impact in initiating and sustaining canker sores by cultivating meaningful connections and learning coping mechanisms.

A substantial body of empirical research supports the effectiveness of stress management strategies in reducing the negative effects of stress on canker sores. Research has indicated that practising mindfulness meditation might lower stress levels in a physiological and psychological way, which may have consequences for oral health. Similarly, studies on progressive muscle relaxation have shown how well it works to reduce symptoms associated with stress and encourage relaxation, which may have an impact on the frequency and severity of canker sores.

Furthermore, methods for cognitive restructuring, supported by cognitive-behavioral theories, have demonstrated potential in modifying how stress is seen and responded to, providing a possible way to break the link between stress and canker sores. A large body of research supports the idea that physical activity can help reduce stress. It highlights the complex effects of physical activity on stress resistance and general well-being, as well as possible implications for oral health outcomes.

Testimonials from people who have included stress management strategies into their daily routines provide as additional evidence of the practical advantages of these strategies in reducing the negative effects of stress on canker sores. Testimonials from individuals demonstrate how mindfulness exercises, gradual muscle relaxation, cognitive restructuring, consistent exercise, and social support can significantly improve resilience and reduce the risk of developing canker sores during times of high stress.

Stress management approaches have a wide range of practical applications in the context of canker sore management, spanning various contexts and scenarios. These tactics provide individuals with actionable strategies to effectively navigate and minimise stress. People can develop a foundation of emotional balance and present-moment awareness by integrating mindfulness meditation into their everyday routines. This could potentially lessen the effect of stress on the occurrence of canker sores. In a similar vein, adding progressive muscle relaxation methods to one's self-care toolkit enables people to take proactive measures to relieve physical strain and stress that worsens canker sores.

By applying cognitive restructuring to stress perception and response patterns, people might possibly change the physiological and emotional cascades linked to the emergence of canker sores by reframing stress-inducing ideas and beliefs. Regular physical exercise not only provides wide-ranging advantages for stress reduction, but it also provides a concrete means of reducing the negative effects of stress on oral health, which may in turn affect the frequency and severity of canker sores.

In addition, developing social support systems and emotional fortitude gives people a strong foundation for managing stress and its possible effects on canker sore treatment. Through the use of constructive relationships and coping mechanisms, people can strengthen their mental health, which may lessen the effect of stress on the development and duration of canker sores.

The methods for stress management that have been outlined provide a comprehensive strategy for reducing the negative effects of stress on oral health as we traverse the complex relationship between stress and canker sore care. These evidence-based practises, which range from mindfulness meditation to physical exercise, give people a comprehensive toolkit to manage stress responses, build resilience, and possibly reduce the impact of stress on the frequency and severity of canker sores. In the sections that follow, we'll go into more detail about how these stress-reduction methods can be included into a comprehensive framework for managing canker sores, with a focus on how they can improve oral mucosal health and emotional wellbeing.

Nutritional Supplements

Addressing dietary inadequacies is essential to the overall care of canker sores since it promotes dental health and lessens the frequency and severity of these oral ulcers. The importance of nutritional supplements in the treatment of canker sores is discussed in this part, along with an examination of the various nutrients and how they contribute to the health of the oral mucosa. This discussion seeks to give a basic understanding of the influence of dietary factors on oral health by analysing the relationship between nutrition and canker sore management. It also provides insights into the possible advantages of nutritional supplementation in reducing the incidence and persistence of canker sores.

The claim that will be discussed in this section concerns the function of dietary supplements in treating particular nutritional deficits associated with the development and aggravation of canker sores. It suggests that by supporting oral mucosal health and lessening the frequency and severity of these oral ulcers, targeted supplementation—which aims to address deficiencies in essential nutrients—can aid in the management of canker sores.

The complex interaction between certain nutrients and the health of the oral mucosa provides the first piece of evidence in support of this claim. More specifically, deficits in minerals like zinc and vitamins like B12, folate, and iron have been linked to a higher risk of developing canker sores. Studies have highlighted the possible effects of these deficits on immunological response, inflammatory responses, and oral mucosal integrity, indicating their involvement in the pathophysiology of canker sores.

Vitamin B12 is an essential nutrient that plays a role in neurological function and DNA synthesis. It has drawn interest in the treatment of canker sores. Because vitamin B12 deficiencies affect mucosal health and immunological responses, they have been connected to oral symptoms, such as mouth ulcers. Likewise, low levels of folate have been linked to a higher incidence of canker sores; folate's function in tissue regeneration and cell division emphasises its importance for maintaining the integrity of the oral mucosa.

Additionally, because iron deficiency anaemia has been linked to recurrent canker sores, iron's potential impact on dental health is highlighted by its vital role in oxygen transport and immunological function. Furthermore, studies have linked the mineral zinc—which is essential for wound healing, immune system function, and inflammatory regulation—to the treatment of canker sores, with the possibility that taking supplements of zinc could shorten the duration and frequency of these lesions.

Rebuttals may focus on the multifaceted character of canker sores, recognising that immunological dysregulation, stress, hormonal fluctuations, and dietary inadequacies can all play significant roles in their aetiology. Furthermore, detractors can draw attention to the possible limits of supplementing in treating nutritional deficiencies, highlighting the necessity of a comprehensive strategy that includes dietary adjustments and lifestyle changes.

In answer to the rebuttals, it is imperative to highlight the relationship between nutritional status and dental health, highlighting the fact that, even though canker sores can result from a variety of causes, treating nutritional deficiencies can be a helpful part of managing them. Furthermore, the explanation can highlight how specific supplements can be used in conjunction with dietary adjustments to address particular deficiencies, which would lead to a more all-encompassing care strategy for canker sores.

Studies explaining the possible advantages of nutritional supplementation in lowering the frequency and severity of canker sores provide more support for the claim. Additional information about the effectiveness of targeted supplementation in reducing the burden of these oral ulcers may come from studies examining the effects of vitamin B complex supplementation, folate, iron, and zinc in people with recurrent canker sores.

In summary, it is impossible to overstate the importance of nutritional supplements in treating certain deficiencies associated with canker sores. Targeted supplementation appears to be a viable strategy for promoting oral health and lowering the incidence and persistence of these oral ulcers because it acknowledges the effects of nutrients like vitamin B12, folate, iron, and zinc on the health of the oral mucosa and their possible roles in the pathophysiology of canker sores. By highlighting the importance of addressing nutritional inadequacies as part of an all-encompassing approach to oral health, this debate prepares the ground for a more nuanced consideration of the possible advantages of nutritional interventions in the holistic management of canker sores.

The Mind-Body Connection

A key idea in comprehending the psychological elements that may influence the onset and healing of canker sores is the mind-body connection. This idea serves as the foundation for understanding the complex interactions that exist between psychological emotions, emotional health, and the physiological processes related to the development and healing of canker sores.

The complex and reciprocal interaction that exists between the mind (including ideas, feelings, and beliefs) and the body is known as the "mind-body connection" (encompassing physical health, physiological processes, and disease states). This link emphasises how psychological variables have a significant impact on the physiological processes of the body and the state of health. The fundamental tenet of the mind-body connection is the recognition that emotional and psychological states can have a real impact on immune system responses, physical processes, and disease susceptibility.

The significant influence of psychological variables on physical health is explained by the mind-body connection, which consists of several essential components. Stress plays a critical role in regulating immunological response and inflammation, which in turn affects the body's vulnerability to a range of diseases, including canker sores. Acute or chronic stress can cause immunological homeostasis to be upset, which can result in dysregulated inflammatory processes that can exacerbate or cause canker sores.

Furthermore, the impact of mental health on physiological functions, such as tissue regeneration and wound healing, is included in the mind-body connection. Optimism and resilience are examples of positive emotional states that have been linked to better immune system performance and better healing results. These findings may have a preventive influence on the severity and duration of canker sores. On the other hand, depressive and anxious states of mind can weaken the immune system and make it more difficult for the body to heal mouth ulcers.

The relationship between mental and physical health served as the foundation for holistic approaches to health and illness in ancient healing traditions, which is where the mind-body link got its start. In order to promote general wellness and treat a variety of illnesses, traditional Chinese medicine and Ayurveda, two ancient healing systems, placed a strong emphasis on the integration of mind, body, and spirit. These traditions promoted psychological equilibrium as the cornerstone of healing, acknowledging the enormous influence that mental states had on physical health.

The biopsychosocial model of health, which recognises the interplay of biological, psychological, and social elements in determining health outcomes, is more broadly consistent with the mind-body connection. This model highlights how psychological moods, behavioural patterns, social circumstances, and biological processes—in addition to genetic predispositions and biological processes—all have an impact on an individual's health status. In this context, the mind-body link highlights the important influence of psychological variables on the development, course, and treatment of canker sores.

Clinical trials and empirical data showing the effect of psychological therapies on health outcomes, like the treatment of oral ulcers, highlight the practical applications of the mind-body connection. Studies have demonstrated that by modifying stress-related immunological responses and inflammatory processes, stress-reduction strategies including mindfulness-based stress reduction and cognitive-behavioral therapy can lessen the intensity and length of canker sores. Similar to this, therapies like relaxation training and resilience-building programmes that work to enhance positive emotional states have been linked to better healing results and a decreased risk of mouth ulcer recurrence.

One of the most prevalent misconceptions about the mind-body link is the oversimplification of its effects, according to which psychological elements are the only ones that affect physical health. While psychological moods can affect physiological processes, it is important to understand that canker sore formation and healing are complicated multifactorial phenomena driven by a complex interplay of genetic, environmental, and behavioural variables. The mind-body link should not be seen as the only factor influencing the development and resolution of oral ulcers, but rather as a major contributing component to the management of canker sores.

In summary, the mind-body link provides a deep understanding of the ways in which psychological variables may influence the onset and course of canker sores. Understanding the complex interactions among mental states, emotional health, and physiological processes, this idea emphasises the need of including psychological considerations in a holistic management strategy for canker sores. Integrating psychological factors into the comprehensive therapy of canker sores is made possible by an understanding of the roles that stress, emotional stability, and psychological interventions play in influencing oral health outcomes.

Lifestyle Modifications for Canker Sore Prevention

The Importance of Oral Hygiene

Clarify the objective the reader will accomplish.

This chapter's objectives are to highlight the vital role that good dental hygiene plays in preventing canker sores and to offer helpful advice for reaching optimal oral health.

List the prerequisites required to accomplish the objective.

Readers will require basic oral hygiene supplies such a toothbrush, toothpaste, dental floss, and mouthwash to accomplish the goal of this chapter. Additionally, it is advised that those with particular oral health difficulties have access to dental care and professional supervision.

Give a snapshot of the steps involved in the process.

Adopting good lifestyle habits, periodic dental checkups, and daily dental care are all important components of maintaining excellent oral hygiene. This comprehensive summary includes the essential elements of dental care that support both general oral health and the avoidance of canker sores.

Break down each part of the process in detail.

1. Apply fluoride toothpaste and a toothbrush with gentle bristles. Brush the tongue and all of the teeth for a minimum of two minutes. Make moderate, circular strokes while keeping an eye on the gum line.

- Every day, wipe the area between your teeth and the gum line to get rid of food particles and plaque that could cause canker sores.

- Rinse your mouth with an alcohol-free mouthwash to eradicate any bacteria that might be causing your oral infections.

2. - Eat a diet high in antioxidants, vitamins, and minerals to promote general oral health. Steer clear of overindulging in spicy or acidic foods since they can irritate the mouth mucosa.

- Sip enough water to keep your mouth wet and encourage the production of saliva, which helps to wash away food particles and maintain the pH balance of your mouth.

3. Limit alcohol intake and abstain from smoking, as these behaviours might irritate oral tissues and jeopardise oral health.

- Be cautious when wearing mouth piercings as they can lead to bacterial infections and mechanical irritation.

4. - Make an appointment for routine dental cleanings to get rid of plaque and tartar accumulation, which can aggravate oral health problems.

- Seek expert guidance and examination to spot any indications of oral health issues, such as canker sores or other lesions.

Give sensible counsel and word of caution.

- If the bristles on your toothbrush start to fray, replace it within three to four months. An outdated toothbrush may exacerbate oral health problems and is less effective at cleaning teeth.

- Avoid using mouthwash excessively as it can upset the natural balance of oral bacteria and cause imbalances in oral health. Instead, use a tongue scraper or your toothbrush to gently clean the surface of your tongue, as bacteria and food debris can accumulate on the tongue and contribute to oral odour and infections.

Describe how to verify successful completion.

Improved oral health indicators, such as a lower frequency of canker sores, healthy gum tissue, and a clean oral environment, can be used to assess whether the oral hygiene techniques described in this chapter have been implemented successfully. Furthermore, routine dental examinations and expert evaluations can confirm the efficacy of the oral hygiene programme.

Provide solutions to common problems that may arise.

It is advised to speak with a dentist if someone continues to have canker sores even when they take great care of their teeth.

Chronic canker sores could be a sign of underlying systemic diseases or particular oral health issues that need for specialist care.

To sum up, good dental hygiene is essential to preventing canker sores and preserving general oral health. People who follow a thorough oral hygiene routine can lower their chance of getting canker sores and promote a healthy oral environment.

Sleep and Canker Sores: The Restorative Connection

There is a complicated and varied relationship between oral health and sleep, and many studies have shown the importance of both quantity and quality of sleep on overall wellbeing. The restorative relationship between sleep and oral health becomes especially important when it comes to managing canker sores. In order to shed light on the ways in which sleep affects dental health and provide guidance on optimising sleep for all-encompassing canker sore care, this chapter will explore the complex interactions that exist between sleep patterns and canker sore prevention and healing.

Canker sore incidence and healing are directly influenced by the quantity and quality of sleep, with sleep pattern disruptions leading to a higher risk of developing canker sores and a slower rate of healing from pre-existing lesions.

Several research works have emphasised the complex connection between immune system performance and sleep, highlighting the significance of sleep in controlling inflammatory and immunological responses. A weakened immune system has been linked to sleep disturbances, especially prolonged sleep deprivation, which increases vulnerability to a number of illnesses, including problems of the oral mucosa such canker sores.

The complex ways in which sleep affects immunological response and inflammation stem from the control of cytokine production, particularly interleukin-1 (IL-1) and tumour necrosis factor alpha (TNF-α), which are essential for regulating immunity of the oral mucosa. It has been demonstrated that sleep deprivation upsets the balance of these cytokines, which increases the inflammatory responses in the oral mucosa and may make canker sores more likely to form and persist.

Furthermore, sleep has a restorative quality that goes beyond immune modulation to include tissue regeneration and repair. The body goes through vital healing processes in the deepest phases of sleep, such as the production of collagen and the release of growth hormone, both of which are necessary for the repair of oral lesions. As a result, insufficient or disturbed sleep can hinder the best healing of oral tissues, extending the course of canker sores and raising the risk of further incidents.

Although there is strong evidence linking sleep to canker sores, it is important to recognise that a person's particular vulnerability to canker sores can vary depending on a number of factors, such as food, dental hygiene habits, and genetic predisposition. Consequently, sleep disturbances may not be the only factor contributing to the formation of canker sores, even though they can worsen their occurrence and healing.

The importance of sleep in managing canker sores is not diminished by the recognition of multiple impacts on susceptibility to canker sores. Instead, it highlights the necessity of an all-encompassing strategy that includes sleep optimization in addition to other preventative measures in order to successfully reduce the incidence and severity of canker sores.

Clinical observations and longitudinal investigations have provided additional support for the link between sleep and canker sores. These research have shown a significant correlation between sleep disturbances and elevated oral mucosal inflammation as well as lesion persistence. The beneficial relationship between sleep and oral health is further shown by the encouraging outcomes of therapies targeted at increasing the quantity and quality of sleep, which have been proven to lessen the frequency and intensity of canker sore episodes.

To sum up, the complex relationship between sleep and canker sores goes beyond a simple correlation. It explores the basic mechanisms by which immune function, inflammatory responses, and tissue repair are modulated by sleep quality and quantity, and how these factors affect the prevention and healing of canker sores. Through an understanding of the healing relationship between sleep and dental health and the application of techniques to improve sleep cycles, people can greatly improve their capacity to control and lessen the effects of canker sores, promoting overall dental health.

Exercise: Boosting Immunity and Reducing Outbreaks

Frequent exercise has been shown to have a host of benefits for mental, emotional, and physical health, making it an essential part of a healthy lifestyle. Regarding the management of canker sores, the impact that exercise may have on immune response and the decrease in breakout frequency offers a strong basis for all-encompassing preventive measures. This chapter will examine the complex relationship between immune modulation and regular physical activity. It will also provide light on the mechanisms by which exercise may reduce the risk of developing canker sores and provide advice on how to incorporate exercise as a preventative measure in a comprehensive approach to managing canker sores.

The main problem here is that canker sores are highly contagious and frequently present as chronic outbreaks or protracted healing times. Phthous ulcers, another name for canker sores, are painful, round or oval lesions that form on the oral mucosa. These lesions cause discomfort and interfere with oral function. The development and duration of canker sores are known to be significantly influenced by immune dysregulation and inflammatory responses, even though their precise origin is still unknown.

Recurrent or untreated canker sores can have a major negative effect on a person's quality of life by causing discomfort when speaking, eating, and taking care of their teeth. Canker sores can also make it harder to practise good oral hygiene, which increases the risk of developing secondary infections or other oral health issues. Moreover, the psychological consequences of recurring canker sores, such as increased tension and worry, can worsen the oral lesions' negative effects on general wellbeing.

Frequent exercise is a possible way to treat the inflammatory reactions and immunological dysregulation linked to canker sores. Participating in regular exercise helps strengthen the immune system, regulate inflammatory processes, and improve overall systemic resilience. These effects may lessen the likelihood of developing canker sores and hasten the healing of current lesions.

Including exercise on a daily basis requires a customised strategy that takes into account personal preferences, physical capabilities, and lifestyle limitations. Programs that include aerobic, resistance, and flexibility training can be customised to meet the needs and fitness levels of a wide range of individuals. In addition, the inclusion of pleasurable physical activities in exercise regimens, including sports, leisure activities, or group fitness courses, may improve adherence to the regimens, supporting long-term immune modulation and possibly preventing canker sores.

Clinical research and physiological studies have provided evidence regarding the potential effectiveness of exercise in immune modulation and the management of canker sores. These studies have shown that regular physical activity can have anti-inflammatory effects, improve immune surveillance, and foster systemic resilience. Further supporting the benefits of exercise in reducing the risk of canker sore susceptibility are long-term studies of participants who exercise regularly, which have shown a decrease in oral mucosal inflammation and a faster healing rate for oral lesions.

Exercise is a potential way to treat canker sores and modulate the immune system, but it's important to recognise that prophylactic measures are complex. Supplementary measures, such as dietary adjustments, stress reduction methods, and improved dental hygiene, could enhance the advantages of physical activity in reducing the risk of canker sores. Consequently, a holistic framework that incorporates several preventative actions may improve the effectiveness of canker sore management techniques in a synergistic manner.

In exploring the possible processes behind the association between exercise and the management of canker sores, it is critical to acknowledge the complex interactions among physical activity, immunological response, and inflammation control. Regular exercise induces a range of systemic adaptations in the body, extending beyond improvements in the cardiovascular and musculoskeletal systems. These adaptations include immunological regulation, stress resilience, and inflammation regulation. Exercise's ability to affect immunological function, inflammatory pathways, and systemic resilience is crucial to understanding how it may affect the management of canker sores. By doing so, it may lessen the risk of developing new lesions and hasten the healing of pre-existing ones.

In summary, the proactive management of canker sores by regular exercise has great potential to influence immunological function, lessen the frequency of outbreaks, and promote overall dental health. Acknowledging the possible impact of exercise on immune control and inflammation management, people can incorporate organised physical activity as a cornerstone of their canker sore prevention tactics, strengthening their resistance to disorders of the oral mucosa and encouraging quicker healing from canker sore bouts. Regular exercise is a proactive and multifaceted approach that complements current preventative measures in a synergistic way, fostering a holistic framework for promoting long-term oral health and mitigating the impact of canker sores. This is particularly important in the pursuit of comprehensive management of canker sores.

Avoiding Oral Trauma

This section's main goal is to offer thorough preventative methods for common oral traumas that can result in canker sores. Readers will be more prepared to limit oral trauma risk and, in turn, lessen the chance that canker sores will form if they are aware of the potential triggers and take proactive actions to avoid them.

People must be willing to take proactive steps to prevent mouth injuries, recognise potential risk factors related to their lifestyle and habits, and comprehend the common causes of oral trauma in order to avoid it. Comprehending the importance of this preventive effort will also benefit from a basic awareness of mouth anatomy and the possible outcomes of oral trauma.

Preventing oral trauma requires a multimodal strategy that includes being aware of possible triggers, changing attitudes and behaviours, and using good mouth hygiene techniques. The stages involved in preventing common forms of oral trauma will be briefly glimpsed in this overview, laying the groundwork for a thorough examination of each element.

1. Recognizing Common Triggers: Recognizing common triggers that might result in injuries within the mouth cavity is the first step towards preventing oral trauma. These triggers can include playing sports that include contact or activities that have a high risk of facial impact, forceful brushing or flossing, eating meals that are too hot or firm, and inadvertently biting one's face or tongue.

2. Changing Routines and Behaviors: After common triggers are recognised, people can concentrate on changing their habits and behaviours to reduce the chance of oral damage. This might be conscious eating to prevent unintentional biting, delicate and deliberate brushing, and extreme caution when handling hot or tough foods. In order to lessen the possibility of oral injuries, people who play contact sports or engage in other activities where there is a

significant risk of facial impact should think about using protection gear, such as mouthguards.

3. Putting Adjudicious Dental Hygiene Into Practice: To prevent oral trauma, it is crucial to employ safe dental care measures in addition to behaviour change. In order to reduce oral tissue irritation, this entails utilising toothbrushes with soft bristles and gentle flossing methods. It also entails practising good oral hygiene to avoid unintentionally damaging the oral mucosa.

- Tip: To lower the danger of thermal damage to the oral tissues, let hot meals or beverages cool to a safe temperature before swallowing them.

- Tip: To prevent potential oral trauma, think about wearing mouthguards when participating in contact sports or other activities where there is a high chance of facial impact.

- Caution: Refrain from vigorous brushing or flossing as this may cause damage to oral tissue and heighten the risk of developing canker sores.

People can keep an eye on their compliance with behaviour modification, oral hygiene routines, and wearing protective gear when engaging in activities that put their mouths in danger to ensure that the techniques for preventing oral trauma are being successfully implemented. Furthermore, the lack of oral trauma cases and a decrease in canker sore cases may function as markers of the effectiveness of these prophylactic actions.

If people find it difficult to change their routines and behaviours to prevent oral trauma, consulting oral health specialists, such dentists or oral hygienists, can offer customised advice and solutions. Furthermore, making use of resources like informational materials and support groups devoted to the prevention of oral injuries can provide insightful information and help in overcoming any obstacles to putting these preventive measures into practise.

In summary, a key element of comprehensive canker sore management is the proactive pursuit of oral injury prevention through the avoidance of common triggers, behaviour and habit adjustment, and application of safe oral care practises. Through the incorporation of these measures into their everyday routines, people can empower themselves to reduce the risk of oral trauma, which in turn lowers the chance of developing canker sores and promotes long-term oral health.

Quitting Smoking: A Path to Better Oral Health

One common practise that has a significant impact on dental health is tobacco use. There is no doubt that using tobacco products—such as smokeless tobacco, cigars, and cigarettes—has a direct correlation to a number of oral health problems, from periodontal disease to oral cancer. But one important but little-studied area of oral health is smoking's effects on the onset and progression of canker sores, or aphthous ulcers. This section explores the complex relationship between smoking and canker sores and discusses the possible advantages of quitting for the purpose of controlling and lowering the frequency of canker sore breakouts.

For those who suffer from recurring breakouts, canker sores—which are defined as painful, round or oval lesions that appear on the soft tissues of the mouth, such as the inner lips, tongue, and cheeks—present a substantial problem. Although the cause of canker sores is complex, new research points to a likely correlation between smoking and an increased risk of developing these incapacitating mouth lesions. Chronic exposure to the carcinogens and nicotine found in tobacco smoke is thought to trigger inflammatory processes in the oral mucosa, which may play a role in the development and persistence of canker sores.

Ignoring the connection between smoking and canker sores can result in a vicious cycle of mouth pain and reduced quality of life for those who have them. In addition to causing excruciating agony and discomfort, canker sores are recurrent and can make it difficult to swallow, speak, or eat. In addition, the psychological anguish brought on by recurrent outbreaks of canker sores can seriously impair a person's general wellbeing, negatively affecting their everyday activities and interpersonal connections.

Giving up smoking is a critical step in reducing the risk of canker sores and promoting better dental health. Giving up tobacco usage may help people reduce the inflammatory mechanisms that underlie the formation of canker sores, which will lessen the frequency and intensity of outbreaks. Additionally, giving up smoking can improve one's overall quality of life and offer a host of holistic health benefits that go beyond oral health.

The application of smoking cessation techniques requires a thorough and customised strategy that takes into account the individual's particular obstacles and driving forces. This could entail seeking out the assistance of medical professionals, participating in behavioural counselling, and making use of pharmaceutical tools like prescription drugs or nicotine replacement therapies. Furthermore, creating a supportive network that includes social, familial, and community networks might help those who are trying to stop smoking remain committed to their long-term sobriety.

Clinical observations and empirical data highlight the revolutionary effect of quitting smoking on oral health outcomes. Research has indicated that persons who successfully quit smoking experience a considerable decrease in the frequency and severity of canker sores. This supports the therapeutic potential of tobacco abstinence in reducing inflammation of the oral mucosa and fostering oral healing. Moreover, quitting smoking leads to a series of systemic health benefits, including enhanced respiratory function, cardiovascular health, and overall longevity, highlighting the long-term advantages of this proactive measure.

Although giving up smoking is the best and most effective intervention for reducing the frequency of canker sores, there are other approaches that can support and strengthen the cessation process. These could involve implementing stress-reduction strategies, altering one's diet to guarantee that one is getting the right amount of nutrients, and implementing dental hygiene routines that support the integrity of one's oral tissue. It is crucial to understand, nevertheless, that these supportive interventions have the greatest effect when combined with quitting smoking, enhancing the combined advantages of a comprehensive approach to oral health.

In summary, giving up smoking is a critical step towards improving oral health and a fundamental component of the all-encompassing treatment of canker sores. Through understanding the complex relationship between smoking and inflammation of the oral mucosa, people can look forward to a life without having to deal with frequent canker sore outbreaks, which will serve as a stepping stone to long-term dental health.

Managing Hormonal Fluctuations

One important, but frequently disregarded, component of canker sore care is the complex relationship between hormone changes and canker sores. Hormonal fluctuations, encompassing variations in levels of progesterone, testosterone, and oestrogen, have a significant impact on the physiological mechanisms that regulate the health of the oral mucosa. In order to demonstrate the critical role that hormone management plays in promoting comprehensive canker sore control, we will unpack the complex relationship that exists between hormonal dynamics and the start, severity, and recurrence of canker sores in this section.

Hormonal fluctuations are a natural part of many physiological states, including puberty, menstruation, pregnancy, and menopause. These fluctuations cause a series of local and systemic actions that have an impact on the mouth cavity. The complex relationship between sex hormones and immune control explains why oral mucosal tissues are more vulnerable to inflammatory and immunological-mediated diseases, which ultimately leads to an increased risk of canker sore development during times of hormonal fluctuations. Notably, variations in progesterone and oestrogen have been linked to immune response modulation, which may exacerbate the inflammatory environment in the oral mucosa and make people more vulnerable to canker sore breakouts. Moreover, testosterone's androgenic effect might possibly play a part in the pathophysiology of canker sores, however additional research is needed to determine exactly what role it plays.

Imagine that a premenopausal lady experiences recurrent bouts of canker sores that coincide with her menstrual cycle's luteal phase, which is marked by elevated progesterone levels. The rise in progesterone that coincides with the fall in oestrogen levels could create an immunological dysregulation milieu that is favourable to the development of canker sores. Through the explanation of these real-world instances, the complex relationship between changes in hormone levels and canker sores is made tangible, highlighting the necessity of customised management approaches to lessen the effects of hormonal dynamics on oral health.

Hormonal variations are complex and require a careful examination of their various consequences for the treatment of canker sores. During the gestational period, which occurs after the menstrual cycle, hormonal surges—mostly those of oestrogen and progesterone—create a dynamic interaction between immune regulation and mouth mucosal health. Moreover, the onset of menopause, which is marked by a decrease in oestrogen levels, may provide a unique set of difficulties with the intensity and susceptibility to canker sores. Through exploring these various viewpoints, we are able to have a comprehensive grasp of the complex effects of hormone changes on the dynamics of canker sores.

The complex association between changes in hormone levels and canker sores is supported by empirical evidence; epidemiological studies have demonstrated that canker sores are more common during specific phases of hormone oscillations. For example, studies have shown that canker sore outbreaks are more common in menstruation individuals throughout the premenstrual and menstrual phases, highlighting the powerful impact of hormone dynamics on oral mucosal integrity. Furthermore, long-term research clarifying the relationship between hormonal treatments and the frequency of canker sores emphasises the significant influence of hormone regulation on dental health results.

The jargon around hormone swings and how they affect dental health needs to be explained in order to promote better understanding. For example, clarifying the notion of dysregulation of the luteal phase and its possible association with worsening of canker sores disentangles the intricate relationship between hormonal dynamics and inflammation of the oral mucosa. We enable readers to understand the fundamental mechanisms coordinating hormonal influences on canker sore dynamics by demystifying such complexities.

Essentially, the complex relationship between changes in hormone levels and canker sores emphasises the need for comprehensive canker sore management plans that include customised treatments that address hormone dynamics. Through understanding the complex effects of hormone increases and decreases on oral mucosal health, people can proactively manage the subtleties of hormonal regulation to prevent canker sore breakouts and promote long-term dental health.

In the next chapters, we will discuss practical methods of controlling hormone fluctuations to lessen the impact of canker sores. These methods include evidence-based therapies and lifestyle changes that align hormonal dynamics with the demands of oral health.

Environmental Factors and Canker Sores

In the field of oral health studies, the role that environmental factors play in the onset and aggravation of canker sores has come under increased scrutiny. Environmental factors are a wide range of factors that can regulate the physiological milieu of the oral mucosa in intricate ways. These factors include climate and pollution levels. This chapter aims to clarify the substantial impact of external factors on oral mucosal integrity and to outline solutions for adaptation and management in the face of environmental difficulties by exploring the complex interplay between environmental determinants and canker sore dynamics.

The main hypothesis supporting this investigation is that environmental factors have a significant impact on the onset and severity of canker sores, and that in order to effectively manage them, it is important to have a thorough grasp of their consequences.

Temperature, humidity, and ultraviolet (UV) radiation are examples of climate variables that are important environmental factors that can have an impact on the health of the oral mucosa. The correlation between climatic conditions and canker sore prevalence has been highlighted by epidemiological studies, wherein specific climatic zones are associated with elevated rates of canker sore outbreaks. Additionally, studies conducted through experimentation have clarified the possible function of ultraviolet light in initiating or intensifying canker sores, supporting the complex relationship between environmental conditions and oral mucosal health.

Variations in humidity and temperature have been shown to upset the oral mucosa's homeostatic equilibrium, which may create an environment that is favourable to the formation of canker sores.

Low humidity levels can have the desiccating effect of drying up the oral mucosa, which puts people at risk for mucosal damage and the subsequent development of canker sores. On the other hand, excessive humidity levels could promote the growth of microorganisms in the mouth, increasing the chance of developing infectious canker sores. Additionally, it has been hypothesised that the immunomodulatory effects of UV radiation cause inflammatory reactions within the oral mucosa, which may exacerbate pre-existing canker sores or encourage the development of new lesions.

While there is increasing evidence linking climate variables to the dynamics of canker sores, there are counterarguments that highlight the complex nature of canker sore aetiology that are worth taking into account. Although environmental influences clearly have an effect on the health of the oral mucosa, their influence may vary depending on an individual's susceptibility and genetic predispositions. Furthermore, the complex interactions between climate factors and other environmental factors require a comprehensive analysis to determine their combined impact on canker sore dynamics.

Despite the fact that the aetiology of canker sores is complex, a significant amount of research has demonstrated a correlation between climatic factors and the prevalence of canker sores. This suggests that customised management approaches that take environmental adaptation into account are necessary. Through recognition of the complex interactions between individual vulnerability and climate, a sophisticated knowledge of the environmental factors influencing canker sores can be used to maximise management strategies.

To further delve into the dynamics of oral health, pollution levels are an important element that should be investigated in relation to the environmental drivers of canker sores. Particulate matter and volatile organic compounds are examples of airborne pollutants that have been linked to systemic and local inflammatory reactions that might impact the oral cavity and perhaps cause or worsen canker sores. The supporting data regarding the detrimental effects of pollution on the integrity of the oral mucosa emphasises the necessity of being alert and adaptable while dealing with environmental issues.

To sum up, the complex relationship between environmental elements and canker sores highlights how important outside factors are in maintaining the health of the oral mucosa. People who understand how pollution and climate change affect the dynamics of canker sores can take proactive steps to reduce the effects of environmental stressors and adjust their lifestyles accordingly. This thorough knowledge of environmental factors opens the door to customised management approaches that balance environmental adaptation with long-term dental health.

Psychological Approaches to Canker Sore Management

Mindfulness and Meditation for Stress Reduction

This chapter's objective is to give a thorough overview of how to use mindfulness and meditation techniques to lessen stress, which has been known to cause canker sores. Through comprehension and application of these strategies, readers will be better equipped to handle stress, which will lower their risk of canker sores.

The only requirement to practising mindfulness and meditation is a willingness to commit time and energy to studying and using these methods. People from various walks of life can participate in these practises because they don't require any specialised equipment or prior knowledge.

Two effective strategies for reducing stress are mindfulness and meditation. This chapter will examine the fundamentals of mindfulness and meditation, as well as the different methods that are used and how they can be used to reduce stress. We will go into great length on how to practise mindfulness and meditation, offer advice and cautions for successful application, and talk about how to confirm that these techniques are beneficial in reducing stress.

1. Understanding Mindfulness:

The practise of mindfulness involves focusing attention on the here and now without passing judgement. It entails being totally conscious of one's thoughts, feelings, physical sensations, and the surroundings around them. Find a peaceful, distraction-free area where you can sit or lie down to start practising mindfulness.

2. Breathing Techniques:

Pay attention to your breathing at first. Notice how every breath feels as you take it in and out. You can just observe the rise and fall of your abdomen or chest, or you can count the breaths you take.

You can help anchor your attention to the present moment and relax your mind by practising the simple act of focusing on your breath.

3. Body Scan Meditation:

A useful technique for cultivating mindfulness is the body scan meditation. Focus on the top of your head first, then slowly work your way down your body, noticing any tense or uncomfortable spots as well as any relaxed spots. This exercise facilitates the release of physical stress and the development of body awareness.

4. Cultivating Mindful Awareness:

Try to incorporate mindfulness into your daily tasks throughout the day. Try to be totally present and alert to the experience, without getting sucked into automatic thoughts or reactions, whether you're eating, strolling, or having a discussion.

5. Introduction to Meditation:

Training the mind to focus and refocus thoughts is part of meditation. As you get more accustomed to the practise, you should progressively extend the length of your meditation sessions. To start, keep them brief—maybe 5 to 10 minutes. Locate a calm and serene setting, take a comfortable seat, and close your eyes.

6. Breath-Focused Meditation:

Breath-focused meditation is among the most widely utilised meditation methods. Take a seat quietly and concentrate on how your breath feels. Gently return your attention, without passing judgement, to the breath whenever your thoughts stray.

7. Loving-Kindness Meditation:

Cultivating love and compassion for oneself and others is the goal of this practise. Start by sending positive vibes your way, and then spread them to friends, family, and even those you might not get along with. Empathy and emotional resilience can be developed through this activity.

8. Yoga and Movement Meditation:

Another effective method for reducing stress is to practise mild yoga or movement-based meditation. These exercises encourage flexibility and relaxation in the body and mind by fusing mindful awareness with physical movement.

- Consistency is key. Aim to practice mindfulness and meditation regularly, ideally daily, to experience the full benefits of these techniques.
- Begin with brief sessions and progressively extend them as you grow more accustomed to the routines.
- Have patience with oneself. During meditation, it's normal for the mind to wander and for stress levels to change. Reject yourself from these events.

Pay attention to your general sense of well-being and your capacity to handle stressors in order to validate the effectiveness of mindfulness and meditation techniques in reducing stress. Check to see if you feel more resilient, at ease, and grounded when faced with difficulties. To monitor your development and consider any shifts in your stress levels over time, keep a journal.

Consider taking a class or using guided meditation recordings if you find it difficult to keep up a regular mindfulness and meditation practise. Establishing a specific area for your practise and scheduling daily time for these activities are also beneficial.

You can develop more serenity, lessen stress, and possibly even prevent canker sores by making mindfulness and meditation routines part of your everyday life. Both meditation and mindfulness are effective strategies for reducing stress and enhancing general wellbeing.

Biofeedback: Controlling the Pain Response

In the last few years, there has been a growing interest in the use of biofeedback therapy for pain management, especially with canker sores. As an intervention, biofeedback presents a viable way for patients to take charge of their pain response, which could result in better pain management for discomfort associated with canker sores. We will explore the fundamentals of biofeedback treatment, how it may be used to control pain, and how it might help people with canker sores in this chapter.

This chapter will focus on the main hypothesis, which is that biofeedback therapy can help patients greatly in controlling their pain response to canker sores, leading to better control over the discomfort that is associated with them.

A non-invasive method called biofeedback therapy uses electronic monitoring to give patients real-time information on physiological processes like skin temperature, heart rate, and muscle tension. Patients can lessen their pain and discomfort by learning to control these body functions and become aware of them.

The manipulation of physiological responses is one of the main methods by which biofeedback operates to control pain. People can learn to actively control their body's functions and experience less pain and related symptoms by getting instant feedback on how their body is functioning. Research has indicated that biofeedback is effective in mitigating pain for a range of ailments, such as musculoskeletal discomfort, headaches, and chronic pain.

Additionally, it has been demonstrated that biofeedback is especially useful in reducing stress, which is a known cause of canker sores. Through the acquisition of physiological response control, individuals can successfully reduce the negative effects of stress on the onset and severity of canker sores.

Although there is a lot of data to support the use of biofeedback in pain management, it is important to be aware of potential objections. Critics contend that the benefits of biofeedback over the long run are unclear and that its effects might be restricted. Furthermore, the cost and accessibility of biofeedback therapy could be obstacles to its widespread use and adoption.

In response to these objections, it is crucial to emphasise that, even though biofeedback therapy might not be a cure-all for all pain-related issues, its potential advantages shouldn't be overlooked when it comes to the treatment of canker sores. Furthermore, biofeedback devices are now more inexpensive and portable thanks to technological improvements, which may help allay some of the accessibility issues surrounding this therapy.

Biofeedback therapy has been shown in recent studies to improve pain perception and pain-related outcomes in a variety of illnesses, including temporomandibular disorders, which are similar to canker sores in terms of pain and discomfort in the mouth. These results lend additional credence to the possible benefits of biofeedback in the therapy of canker sores.

In summary, biofeedback therapy has the potential to be an effective tool for enabling people to take charge of their pain reaction to canker sores. Through the use of real-time physiological feedback, patients can learn how to control their body's reactions, which could result in a decrease in pain perception and better handling of discomfort associated with canker sores. Although additional investigation is necessary to clarify the enduring consequences of biofeedback within this particular setting, the current data highlights its potential as an adjunctive strategy to canker sore treatment.

The Impact of Positive Affirmations

Envision a busy medical facility where individuals from diverse backgrounds seek treatment for a range of health issues. Among the multitude of individuals, Sarah, one patient, sticks out. Her brows knitted due to the agony of a reoccurring canker sore, she walks into the clinic with a noticeable air of misery. Sarah appears uncomfortable on the outside, but her behaviour betrays a deeper discomfort: a lack of self-assurance and a sense of powerlessness in the face of her chronic illness.

Character Depth:

Sarah is a young professional who has a reputation for being smart and hardworking. But her self-esteem has suffered because of the canker sores that haven't gone away. She worries that her coworkers will notice her discomfort or the small lisp from the canker sore, so she feels self-conscious during meetings. Her lively personality is being overshadowed by the emotional weight of this recurrent disease, which is slowly destroying her self-assurance and confidence.

Narrate with Purpose:

Sarah is very nervous as she is led into the consultation room. She takes a seat, and I, Dr. Ankita Kashyap, watch her for a little while. It's clear that her deeper emotional suffering is connected to her physical anguish. This discovery serves as the foundation for our investigation into the effectiveness of positive affirmations in the treatment of canker sores. Our journey goes beyond the domain of physical alleviation to encompass emotional healing and self-empowerment.

Emotional Echo:

Sarah's voice quivers with emotional vulnerability as she discusses the effects of her recurrent canker sores, and her eyes show a mixture of pain and resignation. She talks about cancelled social events, lost opportunities at work, and the ongoing struggle to hide her uneasiness and keep up a brave front. It becomes evident that the psychological impact of canker sores penetrates deeply into one's identity and sense of worth, going much beyond the physical discomfort.

The Unexpected Journey:

It becomes clear from Sarah's storey that canker sore management involves more than just treating the physical symptoms. Emotional turmoil, self-doubt, and a desire for release—not just from the physical pain but also from the psychological weight that comes with it—are hallmarks of the journey. This insight is a sobering reminder of the complex interactions between mental health and physical symptoms that characterise long-term illnesses such as canker sores.

Tie to the Universal:

Sarah's storey is consistent with the widely held belief that long-term illnesses, especially those that show symptoms, can have a substantial negative influence on a person's sense of self and emotional health. The hidden battles people like Sarah fight to keep their lives somewhat normal despite dealing with long-term pain are indicative of a larger storey about human tenacity and the need for holistic treatment—a recovery that takes care of one's body as well as one's spirit.

Entice with Wisdom:

Following Sarah's storey, the use of positive affirmations becomes a ray of hope in the treatment of canker sores. It is a means of accessing inner resilience and a tool that goes beyond the material world to encompass emotional fortitude. The trip that readers will embark on in the upcoming chapters promises to provide insightful understanding of the transformational power of positive affirmations, as well as a road map for recovering confidence and self-worth in the face of canker sore issues.

Introduction to Positive Affirmations:

CBT and mindfulness principles are the foundation of positive affirmations, which are the intentional cultivation of empowering and positive beliefs. This method recognises the complex relationship that exists between ideas, feelings, and actions and suggests that making a conscious effort to steer one's inner monologue in a positive direction can result in significant emotional and psychological changes.

The Power of Self-Talk:

The foundation of positive affirmations is the idea of self-talk, or the internal conversation that moulds our opinions and beliefs about ourselves. People who are managing canker sores frequently struggle with negative self-talk, in which the sores' discomfort and visibility serve as a trigger for feelings of inferiority and self-criticism. Positive affirmations provide a contrast, acting as a purposeful intervention to reframe this mental conversation.

Harnessing Neuroplasticity:

Positive affirmations have the power to transform people because of neuroplasticity, the brain's amazing capacity to rearrange itself by creating new neural connections. People can remodel their neural pathways and cultivate a mindset that is innately more robust, optimistic, and self-assured by regularly participating in positive self-talk. This brain reprogramming has the potential to improve mental environments that support emotional well-being and lessen the psychological effects of long-term ailments like canker sores.

Cognitive Restructuring and Emotional Resilience:

Positive affirmation techniques align with the ideas of cognitive restructuring, which involves people intentionally reframing and challenging unhelpful thought patterns. When it comes to managing canker sores, this approach entails actively battling negative attitudes about one's appearance or perceived limits brought on by the ailment. With time, this intentional reorganisation of mental processes fosters emotional fortitude, enabling people to confront the difficulties presented by canker sores with a revitalised feeling of agency and self-compassion.

The Role of Self-Efficacy:

The idea of self-efficacy, or the conviction that one can exercise control over one's own motivation, conduct, and social environment, is essential to the effectiveness of positive affirmations. When it comes to managing canker sores, fostering a sense of self-efficacy via positive affirmations can cause a significant change in how people view and react to their illness. This agency reduces hopelessness and creates a proactive mindset that supports overall wellbeing by encouraging proactive coping mechanisms.

Clinical Applications and Empirical Evidence:

Studies conducted empirically in the fields of behavioural medicine and psychology have highlighted the observable benefits of positive affirmations in a variety of contexts, from chronic pain management to stress management. Research has demonstrated the beneficial impacts of positive affirmations on developing emotional fortitude, lowering anxiety and depressive symptoms, and improving general psychological health. These results provide a strong basis for investigating the therapeutic uses of positive affirmations in the treatment of canker sores.

The Psychological Burden of Canker Sores:

Painful mouth ulcers known as canker sores frequently coincide with a wide range of psychological stressors. These lesions' appearance, together with the discomfort and possible speech impairment, can cause severe social anxiety and self-consciousness. Furthermore, the repeated nature of canker sores can worsen emotions of frustration and low self-esteem as well as weaken a person's sense of control. This combination of psychological misery and physical suffering emphasises how important it is to treat canker sores holistically, going beyond their physical symptoms.

The Transformative Potential of Positive Affirmations:

In this context, positive affirmations surface as a healing technique that provides those suffering from emotional ulcers with a means of regaining emotional balance and confidence. Through deliberate infusion of affirmations that praise inner strength, self-acceptance, and resilience into their internal dialogue, people can re-calibrate their psychological landscape and cultivate an innately more poised, optimistic, and self-empowered attitude. The possible consequences of this change go beyond simple psychological adjustment; they include a basic reclaiming of identity in the face of persistent discomfort.

The Intersection of Mind and Body:

The foundation of our investigation into the effects of positive affirmations is the symbiotic interaction between the mind and body. It is a recognition that mental health is an essential part of overall health rather than a separate entity. Through cultivating a positive and self-affirming internal environment, people may be able to regulate their physiological reactions to stress, pain, and discomfort. This has significant implications for the treatment of canker sores as well as the overall goal of overall well-being.

Conclusion:

Positive affirmations have a profound effect on canker sore care that goes beyond psychological coping and represents a paradigm leap towards holistic healing. Through the utilisation of positive self-talk, people can undertake a process of self-actualization and emotional fortitude, recovering their autonomy in the face of persistent distress. We will go into more detail on the usefulness of positive affirmations in the context of managing canker sores in the upcoming chapters, providing readers with a road map for incorporating this effective tool into their quest for holistic well-being.

Art Therapy: A Creative Outlet for Healing

The Healing Canvas

The beautiful glow of daylight streams in through huge windows in a calm art therapy studio, giving the space a delicate sheen. The walls are covered in canvases of various sizes, each one bearing witness to the transformational potential of art as a therapeutic and expressive medium. In this peaceful environment, Zach, a patient, uses art therapy to go on a path of self-discovery and emotional healing in order to find relief from the agony of his recurrent canker sores.

Zach, a young professional who is deeply passionate about photography, struggles with the psychological and physical effects of having canker sores on a regular basis. His colourful character, which was before characterised by joy and inventiveness, now struggles with the discomfort and self-consciousness that come with having oral ulcers on a regular basis. I, Dr. Ankita Kashyap, a health and wellness coach, acknowledge the complex relationship between Zach's creative spirit and his battle with chronic pain, which paves the way for a thorough investigation of art therapy as a catalyst for emotional healing.

Zach's life has been overshadowed by the canker sores that never go away, overshadowing the happiness and creative zeal that used to define him. Zach is experiencing self-doubt and mental suffering due to the cyclical nature of his ailment, which has led him to look for ways to find solace that go beyond medical palliation. The task at hand involves treating the severe psychological impact of Zach's recurrent canker sores and reestablishing his internal balance using a body-mind-spirit holistic approach.

A moving and multifaceted method for healing the psychological toll that chronic canker sores take is art therapy. People such as Zach are able to access deeper levels of their psyche by externalising their internal challenges, feelings, and goals through visual creativity, which transcends the limitations of verbal expression. Zach is encouraged to transform his canker sore experiences into vivid, expressive artwork in the studio's healing cocoon, which promotes contemplation, release, and emotional catharsis.

Zach's emotional landscape undergoes a noticeable transformation as he immerses himself in the field of art therapy. He conveys the subtleties of his experience with recurrent canker sores through his artwork, capturing moments of resiliency, fragility, and calm strength in the vivid colours and expressive brushstrokes of his works. Zach's behaviour changes slightly with every session, peeling away layers of mental pain to reveal a developing sense of inner serenity, fortitude, and self-acceptance that goes beyond his physical anguish.

Zach's involvement with art therapy is a compelling case study that highlights the important relationship between creativity and emotional recovery. It emphasises how artistic expression may go beyond language barriers and explore the depths of a person's emotional environment, providing a healing path for people dealing with chronic illnesses like canker sores. Zach's journey also encourages reflection on the universal potential of art therapy as a holistic approach that supports self-discovery, emotional release, and the restoration of inner balance in the face of persistent distress.

Zach's storey is accompanied by powerful images that capture his artistic expressions and provide a moving look into the deep emotional undercurrents that permeate his work. Readers can better understand the emotional resonance of art therapy as a tool for navigating the complexities of chronic conditions by using these visual aids, which go beyond verbal articulation to access the unfiltered, raw emotions that serve as the foundation for the process of healing and self-discovery.

Zach's art therapy experience is a microcosm of the larger storey of integrative medicine and wellbeing. It emphasises how important it is to welcome a range of approaches that go beyond traditional medical treatments, realising the inextricable relationship between mental health, artistic expression, and the treatment of long-term illnesses. Through the incorporation of art therapy into the care of canker sores, we shed light on the transformational power of holistic healing that takes into account both emotional and physical aspects.

As we watch Zach's journey of transformation via art therapy, an idea nags at us: How might the expressive domains of music, dance, and art function as pathways for healing and emotional release within the maze-like world of chronic pain? This question invites readers to consider the various ways that art can weave a tapestry of emotional healing among the difficulties presented by chronic diseases, and it also calls us to delve deeper into the relationship between creative expression and holistic wellness.

In the next few chapters, we will take an in-depth look at a variety of therapeutic approaches that come together to create a comprehensive guide for managing canker sores. This guide goes beyond traditional medical interventions to include art therapy, mindfulness exercises, dietary changes, and building emotional fortitude. By working together, we will be able to reveal the many facets of holistic wellbeing and provide readers with a clear road map for negotiating the complex world of persistent suffering with dignity, fortitude, and deep self-empowerment.

Journaling for Emotional Release and Tracking

This section aims to clarify the significant advantages of journaling as a tracking tool for canker sore outbreaks and as a way to vent during the uncomfortable periods. By exploring the nuances of journaling, we hope to provide readers a thorough grasp of how this practise can be a game-changer in the treatment of persistent canker sores, promoting emotional healing and offering insightful information to medical professionals.

The only necessary precondition to journaling for monitoring and releasing emotions is the desire to reflect on and record one's experiences. Although the main tool for keeping track of thoughts and feelings can be a physical notebook or a digital platform like a computer or smartphone, the most important thing is that the person making the effort to participate in the process as a way to express their feelings and reflect on themselves.

Emotional catharsis and factual documentation are two aspects of the complex process that is journaling for monitoring and emotional release. Through this activity, people are able to communicate their feelings about breakouts of canker sores, which promotes a sense of release and self-expression. At the same time, it makes it possible to monitor canker sore incidents systematically, which advances our knowledge of the patterns and possible causes of these episodes.

There are a number of connected phases involved in journaling for emotional release and tracking, and each one is important for developing emotional resilience and improving self-awareness in the face of chronic canker sore issues.

1. The first step in the trip is to start journaling, which encourages people to set aside specific time for reflection and

emotional writing. This could involve journaling every day to record ideas and feelings, especially during canker sore breakouts, or it could involve keeping an ongoing diary to monitor the frequency and severity of these episodes.

2. Expressing one's feelings about canker sore eruptions is a crucial part of the journaling process. This could entail documenting the discomfort felt physically during these periods in addition to exploring the emotional fallout, including annoyance, worry, or self-consciousness. Through the process of writing in a diary, people can release the psychological burden that comes with canker sore incidents, leading to a feeling of emotional catharsis and release.

3. Concurrently, journaling is an essential tool for monitoring the development and occurrence of canker sores. People are advised to document the beginning of every episode, the length of time the sore lasted, any accompanying symptoms, and any possible exacerbating or trigger events. The thorough documentation makes it easier to identify patterns and triggers, which provides individuals and healthcare practitioners with useful information to help them develop customised management strategies.

4. By reflecting and analysing diary entries on a regular basis, people can identify trends, stressors, and emotional reactions related to canker sore outbreaks. This stage provides an opportunity for self-reflection, as participants are asked to determine any possible associations between emotional states, dietary practises, stress levels, and the development of canker sores. By means of this introspective process, people acquire an enhanced consciousness of the relationship between their emotional state and the occurrence of mouth ulcers, therefore enabling them to take proactive measures to address these occurrences. The importance of constancy in keeping a journal for tracking and emotional release cannot be overstated. Urge them to develop a committed journaling practise regardless of how intense their emotions are or how often they get canker sores.

Regular recording enhances the value of journaling in identifying trends and promoting emotional release. Insist that people accept raw self-expression in their diaries and reassure them that this is a nonjudgmental activity. People must have the confidence to express their feelings honestly and without hesitation or self-censorship.

- Encourage them to enter the reflective analysis phase with an open mind and receptive heart. To promote a spirit of empirical inquiry and self-discovery, encourage them to investigate possible links between emotional states, lifestyle factors, and canker sore outbreaks without preconceived assumptions.

- Although writing can be a means of facilitating emotional release, it is imperative to advise people not to focus only on upsetting feelings when journaling. Urge them to look for a fair representation of their experiences that includes resiliency moments, coping mechanisms, and emotional fortitude in the face of the difficulties presented by canker sores.

The concrete advantages that those who journal for emotional release and tracking can attest to verify the effectiveness of this activity. This includes less emotional discomfort during episodes of canker sores, increased awareness of possible triggers, and the development of proactive care plans based on the knowledge gained from journaling.

In conclusion, for those struggling with chronic canker sores, journaling as a means of emotional release and tracking offers a transforming approach. Through the process of charting the development of mouth ulcers, articulating their emotional responses, and engaging in reflective analysis, people gain the ability to manage their canker sores with grace, resilience, and increased self-awareness. By incorporating journaling into the larger canker sore mastery blueprint, we shed light on the fundamental relationship between emotional health and managing chronic conditions. This provides readers with a comprehensive framework for promoting emotional healing and knowledgeable self-empowerment while navigating the difficulties presented by recurring canker sores.

Self-Care and Home Remedies

Over-the-Counter Solutions

I. When it comes to the treatment of canker sores, over-the-counter (OTC) products are easily available and practical options for people who want to alleviate the pain and discomfort that these mouth ulcers cause. The goal of this in-depth analysis of over-the-counter remedies is to offer a full assessment of their efficacy by illuminating their modes of action, supporting data, and useful implications. We want to provide readers with the information they need to treat their canker sores wisely, so we've explored the subtleties of each therapy.

II. III. a. b. Because hydrogen peroxide is a well-known antiseptic agent and can help clean the afflicted region and encourage healing, it is frequently used in the therapy of canker sores. Hydrogen peroxide can be used as a mouthwash to help remove debris from the canker sore and lower the bacterial burden when diluted properly.

c. Hydrogen peroxide has been shown in numerous trials to be effective in lessening the length and intensity of canker sores. Furthermore, a great deal of people have observed that using hydrogen peroxide rinses has expedited recovery and relieved suffering.

d. People can use this treatment by combining equal parts water and 3 percent hydrogen peroxide, then swishing the mixture about in their mouths for 30 seconds before spitting it out. This is a useful and easily attainable method of treating canker sores, and it can be done up to four times a day.

IV.

Following the exploration of hydrogen peroxide rinse, we turn our attention to another widely used OTC solution, benzocaine gel.

b.

b. A local anaesthetic called benzocaine works by numbing the affected area when applied, providing momentary respite from the agony and suffering brought on by canker sores. In order to temporarily relieve the sensations of soreness and irritation, it works by preventing pain signals from the affected place from reaching the brain.

c. Benzocaine gel is a well-liked option for people looking for quick relief from the agony of canker sores because clinical trials and customer reviews have repeatedly shown how quickly it relieves pain.

d. To make good use of benzocaine gel, people should dab a little bit of it on the canker sore with a cotton swab, covering the surrounding region as well to ease any pain. Even though this remedy provides short-term relief, it's crucial to follow the suggested application frequency to prevent any negative side effects.

V.

Transitioning from benzocaine gel, we delve into the realm of oral pain relief patches.

b.

b. Oral pain patches offer a focused and prolonged supply of pain relief to the affected location. These patches frequently contain active substances like menthol or benzocaine. These patches adhere to the interior of the mouth to provide continuous pain relief, enabling people to resume their everyday activities without being impeded by the agony of canker sores.

c. Dental pain treatment patches have been shown to provide long-lasting pain relief in clinical trials; users have reported notable gains in their ability to eat, speak, and practise good oral hygiene. The continuous and dependable relief of canker sore symptoms is guaranteed by the localised and controlled release of active substances.

d. Applying oral pain treatment patches entails sticking the patch straight to the afflicted area and making sure it stays there for the prescribed amount of time. With the least amount of interference to their everyday lives, people can now control their canker sores thanks to this easy-to-use and covert treatment.

VI.
Shifting our focus to mouthwashes and rinses, we explore their role in canker sore management.

b.

b. Antimicrobials, anti-inflammatory chemicals, and calming agents are frequently found in mouthwashes and rinses designed especially for the treatment of canker sores. These treatments aid in the general alleviation and quick healing of canker sores by cleaning the afflicted region, lowering inflammation, and producing a calming effect.

c. Research has shown that using specific mouthwashes and rinses might lessen the duration and severity of canker sores. Users have reported feeling relieved and their ability to restore oral function has been restored. These remedies' specific activity at the site of the canker sore encourages a healing environment.

d. To clean the mouth cavity and encourage the healing of canker sores, people can use mouthwashes and rinses as prescribed as part of their oral hygiene routine. Individuals can proactively manage and decrease the impact of canker sores on their oral health by including these treatments into their everyday routine.

VII. Moving on to the topic of oral analgesic gels and liquids, we examine their potential for the treatment of canker sores.

b. b. By numbing the afflicted area and lessening pain perception, oral analgesic gels and liquids with active substances like phenol or lidocaine provide focused relief from canker sore pain. Their mixture relieves the pain and irritation brought on by canker sores with ease of administration and quick alleviation.

c. Clinical research has proven the effectiveness of oral analgesic gels and liquids in delivering quick and long-lasting pain relief, allowing people to resume their regular activities with little difficulty. Testimonials from users have confirmed that they value the quick relief that these over-the-counter remedies provide.

d. When applying oral analgesic gels and liquids, make sure to thoroughly cover the surrounding region for complete relief by carefully dispense the substance into a cotton swab or directly onto the canker sore. People can effectively reduce the discomfort associated with canker sores by using the advantages of these treatments by according to the suggested application instructions.

VIII. To sum up, people have a variety of options to suit their individual needs and preferences thanks to the availability of over-the-counter (OTC) canker sore care remedies. People can decide which course of action is best for managing and relieving their canker sores by critically analysing the mechanisms of action, empirical data, and useful uses of these remedies. By incorporating over-the-counter medications into one's regimen for managing canker sores, people can take proactive measures to address the symptoms and consequences of these oral ulcers, which in turn promotes a more comfortable and functional oral environment.

Rinses and Washes

This chapter's objective is to offer comprehensive instructions for making homemade mouthwashes that relieve canker sores. Readers will be prepared to construct simple and efficient therapies for the management of canker sores by knowing the qualities of various natural components and their capacity to ease suffering.

People will need basic household tools like baking soda, salt, and water, as well as natural substances like sage, chamomile, and aloe vera, to make the homemade mouth rinses. To guarantee precise preparation, you'll also need a measuring spoon and a clean storage container.

A cheap and natural way to treat canker sores is with homemade mouth rinses. Through the utilisation of particular substances with calming and antibacterial qualities, these rinses seek to lessen inflammation, ease discomfort, and facilitate the healing process of canker sores.

a. Aloe vera, well known for its restorative and anti-inflammatory qualities, can be used to make a calming mouthwash to treat canker sores. An important component of this DIY rinse is the gel that is taken from the aloe vera plant. These components help to promote tissue repair and reduce discomfort.

One teaspoon fresh aloe vera gel and one cup lukewarm water can be used to make an aloe vera mouth rinse. Before spitting out, this solution can be spun about in the mouth for thirty seconds. To continue providing relief, this rinse can be applied several times a day.

b. Chamomile, which has antibacterial and anti-inflammatory qualities, can be a calming ingredient in a homemade mouthwash for the treatment of canker sores. The natural substances included in chamomile help to relieve pain, lessen swelling, and speed up the healing process for mouth ulcers.

One chamomile tea bag can be steeped in one cup of hot water for ten minutes, then allowed to cool before using as a mouth rinse. You can use the cooled chamomile tea as a mouthwash by swishing it about in your mouth for 30 seconds and then spitting it out. To keep this rinse's calming effects going, use it several times during the day.

c. Sage, which has antibacterial and anti-inflammatory qualities, can be used to a DIY mouthwash to help treat canker sores. Sage's natural ingredients fight oral bacteria, ease inflammation, and speed up the healing process for canker sores.

One tablespoon of dried sage can be steeped for fifteen minutes in one cup of hot water to make a sage mouth rinse. Let the mixture cool before using. You can use the cooled sage infusion as a mouthwash by swishing it about in your mouth for 30 seconds and then spitting it out. To maximise the therapeutic benefits of this rinse, use it many times a day.

The effectiveness of the homemade mouth rinses depends on the use of high-quality, fresh natural components; people who have a history of sensitivities to any particular ingredient should take caution and seek medical advice before using these rinses.

- When treating severe or recurrent canker sores, these DIY rinses provide some natural relief, but they shouldn't be used in place of expert medical counsel and care.

Reduction of swelling, improvement in the healing of the oral ulcers, and relief from the pain associated with canker sores are indicators that the DIY mouth rinses were successful. By keeping a close eye on their symptoms and documenting any improvement in their health, users can evaluate the efficiency of the rinses.

If there is little to no relief or any negative responses, people should stop using the DIY mouth rinses and consult a medical expert. For full care of severe or recurring canker sores, it is imperative to find and treat any underlying causes.

Finally, the homemade mouthwash recipes in this chapter provide people with an easy-to-use, all-natural way to treat canker sores. People can make powerful rinses to ease pain, encourage healing, and create a more comfortable oral environment by utilising the therapeutic qualities of aloe vera, chamomile, and sage. Including these DIY mouthwashes in your regimen for managing canker sores gives people the ability to take control of the signs and consequences of these oral ulcers and promote better oral health.

Topical Applications

Topical treatments are essential for the treatment of canker sores because they provide focused pain relief and aid in the healing process. This chapter will look at a variety of over-the-counter and natural topical treatments that have shown promise in reducing discomfort and encouraging the healing of canker sores. Through an exploration of the workings, characteristics, and real-world uses of various topical medicines, readers will obtain important knowledge on how to include these treatments into their care plans for canker sores.

    a. The healing of wounds, antibacterial, and anti-inflammatory qualities of honey have all been acknowledged. It is a potential topical therapy for the treatment of canker sores because of these qualities. Because honey has a high sugar content, it fosters a moist wound healing environment while inhibiting the growth of bacteria. Additionally, honey has ingredients that help to lessen inflammation and hasten the healing of canker sores.

    Studies have demonstrated the potential of honey in wound healing, demonstrating how it can speed up the healing process and lessen pain. Furthermore, anecdotal data from those who have experienced canker sores has confirmed the calming and restorative properties of immediately applying honey to mouth ulcers.

    Honey can be applied topically to control canker sores by immediately applying a little amount of raw, unprocessed honey to the afflicted region. You can use honey's healing powers to relieve and treat canker sores by doing this several times a day.

    As we go on to the next topical application, it's critical to take into account coconut oil's numerous advantages for the treatment of canker sores.

    b. Because of its strong antibacterial and anti-inflammatory qualities, coconut oil is a useful topical treatment for canker sores.

Because lauric acid in coconut oil has antimicrobial properties against a range of pathogens, it may help lower the number of oral microorganisms linked to canker sores. Moreover, using coconut oil to the affected area can help to moisturise it, encourage tissue repair, and ease discomfort.

Research has demonstrated that coconut oil has antibacterial properties that make it effective against oral bacteria and fungus. Furthermore, people who have included coconut oil into their regimen for treating canker sores have experienced less discomfort and faster oral ulcer healing.

People can massage a tiny quantity of organic, virgin coconut oil directly onto the sore spot in order to relieve their canker sores. To take use of coconut oil's antibacterial and calming qualities for the treatment of canker sores, repeat this several times a day.

Now that we have moved on to the next topical treatment, licorice gel, it is important to investigate its potential for delivering focused relief for canker sores.

c. The root of the licorice plant yields licorice gel, which is made up of bioactive substances such glycyrrhizin and flavonoids with antiviral, anti-inflammatory, and immunomodulatory qualities. Because of its ability to lower inflammation, stop the growth of oral infections, and alter the immune system in the oral cavity, licorice gel is a potent topical treatment for canker sores.

Studies have shown that licorice gel has antiviral and anti-inflammatory properties, suggesting that it may be used to reduce oral inflammation and encourage tissue repair. In addition, people who have used licorice gel to treat canker sores have reported less discomfort and faster healing of mouth ulcers.

People can apply licorice gel directly to the problematic area, using a small amount of the gel to relieve canker sores. Licorice gel's anti-inflammatory and immunomodulatory qualities can be utilised for the treatment of canker sores by performing this several times daily.

As we go on to the next topical treatment, benzocaine-based medicines, it is important to investigate their potential for canker sore pain alleviation and regional anaesthetic.

d. A typical ingredient in over-the-counter medications intended to relieve oral pain, particularly the discomfort associated with canker sores, is benzocaine, a local anaesthetic. By preventing nerve impulses from entering the body, benzocaine relieves canker sore pain and discomfort momentarily. This makes topical applications containing benzocaine a practical and efficient way to treat pain associated with canker sores.

Studies on patients with a variety of oral diseases, including canker sores, have shown that benzocaine is effective in reducing discomfort and promoting regional anaesthetic. Furthermore, people who have taken medications containing benzocaine have reported a notable decrease in the pain and discomfort related to mouth ulcers.

Applying a tiny amount of benzocaine-based products directly to the affected area and following the manufacturer's instructions for dosage and application frequency is one way to use them for relief from canker sores. Following the suggested usage guidelines is crucial to ensuring canker sore pain alleviation that is both safe and effective.

Moving on to the last topical treatment, hydrogen peroxide rinse, it is important to investigate its potential for encouraging good oral hygiene and supporting the treatment of canker sores.

e. Because of its antibacterial qualities, hydrogen peroxide can be a useful topical treatment for canker sores. Hydrogen peroxide can successfully lower oral bacteria and promote the healing of canker sores when diluted to a safe quantity. Furthermore, hydrogen peroxide's bubbling action can help to promote dental hygiene and clean the affected area.

Scientific studies have proven hydrogen peroxide's antibacterial effectiveness, highlighting its capacity to lower oral bacterial load and promote oral ulcer healing. In addition, people who have included hydrogen peroxide rinses in their dental hygiene regimen have reported faster healing times for canker sores.

In order to apply hydrogen peroxide topically for the treatment of canker sores, people can make a diluted hydrogen peroxide rinse by combining equal parts water and 3 percent hydrogen peroxide. You can briefly swirl this solution around in your mouth before spitting it out. To guarantee the safe and efficient administration of hydrogen peroxide for the treatment of canker sores, it is imperative to adhere to the suggested dilution and dosage guidelines.

To sum up, this chapter's wide range of topical applications provides people with a comprehensive toolkit for handling canker sosores. Readers can make well-informed decisions about the incorporation of honey, coconut oil, licorice gel, benzocaine-based treatments, and hydrogen peroxide rinse into their regimen for managing canker sores by being aware of the mechanisms, characteristics, and real-world uses of these therapies. These topical treatments not only offer focused relief from the pain and discomfort associated with canker sores, but they also aid in the healing of oral ulcers, promoting better oral health and improving the general wellbeing of those who deal with canker sores.

Managing Pain and Discomfort

Canker sores, also known as aphthous ulcers, are a common oral condition that results in painful, spherical or oval lesions on the mucous membranes of the mouth. These ulcers can cause severe discomfort and make it difficult to perform simple oral functions like eating, speaking, and cleaning your teeth. A person's quality of life may be significantly impacted by canker sore pain and discomfort, which can make daily tasks challenging and psychologically distressing.

The treatment of canker sore pain and discomfort is the primary concern here. Because of the excruciating pain that is experienced when eating, drinking, and speaking as well as the continuous discomfort that these oral ulcers bring, effective strategies for easing these symptoms and enhancing the overall wellbeing of those who have canker sores are needed.

If the pain and discomfort caused by canker sores are not adequately handled, people may find it difficult to consume vital nutrients, drink plenty of water, and interact with others. Additionally, the continuous discomfort could make stress and anxiety worse, which could be detrimental to one's emotional and mental well-being. Furthermore, discomfort that is left untreated might prevent canker sores from healing on their own, lengthening the ulcer's life and aggravating its overall consequences on oral health.

The pain and discomfort caused by canker sores can be reduced with a comprehensive plan that includes topical treatments, dental hygiene, and lifestyle modifications. By applying targeted pain and discomfort management approaches, people can reduce the symptoms of canker sores and expedite the healing process, both of which will improve their quality of life in the long run.

Applying pain and discomfort management strategies involves changing one's lifestyle to lessen triggers and improve overall health, maintaining the highest standards of oral cleanliness to promote the healing of canker sores, and using topical therapies to provide focused relief.

Carefully implementing comprehensive pain and discomfort management techniques can help people experience reduced pain and discomfort from canker sores, quicker healing from mouth ulcers, and an overall improvement in their dental health and quality of life.

While topical therapies for pain and suffering are the main emphasis of this chapter, the management of canker sores can be greatly improved by utilising other strategies such as dietary modifications, stress-reduction techniques, and professional interventions.

We will now focus on the use of pain and discomfort management strategies as we carry out our inquiry into the treatment of canker sores. We will specifically talk about using topical treatments to lessen canker sore-related symptoms.

Topical Applications for Pain and Discourage Management

Since topical therapies offer targeted relief and facilitate the healing process of these oral ulcers, they are an indispensable component of canker sore management. By understanding the roles, traits, and practical applications of various topical treatments, individuals can effectively reduce the pain and suffering associated with canker sores, hastening the healing process and improving oral health in general.

For canker sores to provide focused pain and discomfort alleviation, topical therapies are crucial. These therapies can release medicinal compounds that help lessen symptoms and promote mouth ulcer healing by coming into close touch with the affected area. One proactive approach to treating canker sores is to use topical therapies, which will address the immediate symptoms and encourage the oral mucosa's natural healing process.

a. Chamomile is an effective topical treatment for canker sore pain and discomfort because of its anti-inflammatory and calming qualities. Applying a compress made of chamomile can have a mild, relaxing impact on the affected area, which may help to lessen pain and inflammation related to mouth ulcers.

Studies have demonstrated that chamomile has anti-inflammatory properties, which enable it to reduce inflammation of the oral mucosa and offer treatment to those who suffer from canker sores. Moreover, anecdotal data from people who have applied chamomile compresses has confirmed the calming and pain-relieving properties on mouth ulcers.

People can soak chamomile tea bags in hot water, let them cool, and then apply the compress directly to the affected area for several minutes to relieve pain and discomfort associated with canker sores. To use chamomile's calming and anti-inflammatory qualities to treat canker sores, repeat this several times a day.

As we go on to the next topical remedy, aloe vera gel, we must investigate its potential for canker sore cooling and healing properties.

b. Aloe vera gel is well known for its ability to soothe and repair wounds, which makes it a useful topical treatment for canker sore pain. Applying aloe vera gel to the oral ulcers helps create a protective and calming barrier, which may lessen discomfort and encourage tissue healing.

Aloe vera gel's capacity to cure wounds has been demonstrated by scientific studies, which also highlight the gel's capacity to hasten the healing of oral mucosal tissues and reduce oral ulcer pain. Moreover, people who have used aloe vera gel in their regimen for treating canker sores have experienced less discomfort and faster oral ulcer healing.

A tiny amount of premium aloe vera gel can be immediately applied to the affected area to relieve canker sores, being sure to create a protective covering over the mouth ulcers. To utilise aloe vera gel's cooling and healing qualities for the treatment of canker sores, repeat this several times a day.

Let's move on to the next topical remedy, vitamin E oil. It's important to investigate how this oil might help with tissue healing and canker sore relief.

c. Because of its anti-inflammatory and tissue-repairing qualities, vitamin E oil is a useful topical treatment for canker sore pain and discomfort. By lowering discomfort and hastening tissue repair, using vitamin E oil can aid in the oral ulcer's natural healing process.

Studies have demonstrated the antioxidant capacity of vitamin E oil and demonstrated how it can help people with canker sores by facilitating the healing of oral mucosal tissues. Furthermore, people who have used vitamin E oil to treat canker sores have reported less discomfort and faster healing of mouth ulcers.

Applying a small amount of vitamin E oil straight to the affected area and gently massaging it into the oral ulcers is one way that people might use it to relieve canker sores. To use vitamin E oil's antioxidant and tissue-repairing qualities to treat canker sores, repeat this several times a day.

Moving on to the next topical medication, mouthwash containing sage, we must investigate its ability to treat canker sores by acting as an antibacterial and an anti-inflammatory.

d. Sage is a useful topical treatment for canker sore pain and discomfort because of its antibacterial and anti-inflammatory qualities. By using a sage mouthwash, you might potentially reduce inflammation and offer treatment to those who suffer from oral ulcers by creating an environment that hinders the formation of oral germs.

Sage has been shown in research to have antibacterial and anti-inflammatory properties, which suggests that it may help maintain dental health and reduce pain from canker sores. Additionally, people who have included sage mouthwash in their regimen for treating canker sores have reported feeling less discomfort and having better dental hygiene.

In order to make a sage mouthwash that relieves canker sores, people can soak dried sage leaves in boiling water to make a herbal infusion, let it cool, and then apply the mouthwash, making sure it gets to the sore spot. To use sage's antibacterial and anti-inflammatory qualities to treat canker sores, repeat this several times a day.

As we go on to the last topical remedy, clove oil, it is important to investigate its potential for canker sore analgesic and antibacterial properties.

e. Strong analgesic and antibacterial qualities of clove oil make it an effective topical treatment for canker sore pain and discomfort. Clove oil application has the ability to reduce discomfort and accelerate the healing of oral ulcers by inhibiting the growth of oral infections and providing regional pain relief.

Healing Boosters

As we delve further into the practise of comprehensive canker sore therapy, it becomes imperative to look into methods for accelerating the healing of these mouth ulcers. Healing a canker sore faster not only relieves the pain and discomfort associated with it, but it also speeds up the restoration of general oral health and wellness. This chapter will offer a detailed explanation of each healing booster, including its mechanics, applications, and potential impact on the natural healing process of canker sores.

The list of carefully chosen therapeutic supplements that might hasten the healing of canker sores is as follows:

a. Propolis is a resinous material that bees gather from sap flows, tree buds, and other botanical sources. It has amazing wound-healing, antibacterial, and anti-inflammatory qualities. Flavonoids, phenolic compounds, and terpenes are some of its constituents, which enhance its medicinal value in the treatment of canker sores. When applied topically, propolis extract forms a barrier that protects the ulcer and speeds up healing by encouraging tissue repair and stifling microbial growth.

Propolis's antibacterial and anti-inflammatory properties have been shown in clinical trials to be effective in hastening the healing of mouth ulcers. Moreover, people who have used propolis extract to treat canker sores have experienced quicker healing times and less discomfort.

Applying a tiny amount of propolis extract directly to the afflicted region with a clean cotton swab can help people take advantage of the healing potential of propolis extract for canker sore care. This treatment can be used several times a day to offer long-term therapeutic assistance for the canker sores' natural healing process.

Moving on to the next healing enhancer, honey and turmeric, it is critical to investigate their synergistic benefits in aiding in the healing of canker sores.

b. Turmeric and honey combined form a strong paste that has significant antibacterial, anti-inflammatory, and wound-healing qualities. Curcumin, a molecule with anti-inflammatory and antioxidative effects, is present in turmeric, which works in concert with honey, which is recognised for its antibacterial action and capacity to foster an environment that is favourable for tissue healing. This combination promotes the restoration of dental health by accelerating the healing process and relieving the discomfort brought on by canker sores.

Studies have demonstrated the antibacterial and anti-inflammatory properties of turmeric and honey, as well as their capacity to hasten the healing of mouth ulcers. Furthermore, people who have managed their canker sores with the honey and turmeric paste have experienced faster healing times and better pain relief.

A spoonful of raw, organic honey and a pinch of turmeric powder can be combined to make a smooth, uniform paste that people can use to relieve canker sores. After that, you can apply this paste directly to the afflicted area, making sure to fully cover the mouth ulcers. To take advantage of the complementary therapeutic properties of turmeric and honey for the treatment of canker sores, repeat the application several times a day.

As we move on to the next healing enhancer, zinc supplementation, it is important to examine how it can aid in tissue mending and lessen canker sore symptoms.

c. Zinc, an important mineral with a variety of physiological uses, is crucial for wound healing, tissue repair, and immune system function. Its antibacterial action, cell proliferation, and inflammatory modulation make it an important healing enhancer for the treatment of canker sores. Zinc supplements not only help the body's defence mechanisms but also hasten oral ulcer healing, which may shorten the time and lessen the severity of canker sores.

Clinical research has proven that zinc supplements are effective in helping mouth ulcers heal, highlighting the mineral's function in boosting immune responses and tissue healing mechanisms. In addition, people who have used zinc supplements in their regimen for treating canker sores have experienced quicker healing rates and fewer oral ulcer recurrences.

People who want to relieve their canker sores may want to think about including foods high in zinc, like nuts, seeds, legumes, and lean meats, in their diet. As an alternative, zinc supplements can be taken to guarantee sufficient intake for promoting the healing process of canker sores, after consulting with a medical practitioner.

As we go on to the next healing enhancer, licorice paste, we must investigate its ability to treat canker sores by acting as an antibacterial and reducing inflammation.

d. The root of the Glycyrrhiza glabra plant yields licorice, which is a plant that includes bioactive substances including flavonoids and glycyrrhizin that have strong antibacterial, anti-inflammatory, and wound-healing qualities. Licorice, when made into a paste and applied externally, soothes the mouth ulcers, lowers inflammation, and stops the growth of germs, creating an environment that promotes faster recovery.

Studies have demonstrated the anti-inflammatory and antibacterial properties of licorice, demonstrating how well it can aid in the healing of oral ulcers and reduce pain that goes along with them. Furthermore, people who have used licorice paste to treat canker sores have reported better symptom relief and faster healing.

People can make licorice paste to relieve canker sores by combining licorice root powder with a tiny amount of water to create a paste-like consistency. The oral ulcers can be completely covered by applying this paste directly to the affected area. The anti-inflammatory and antibacterial qualities of licorice can be used to treat canker sores by applying the mixture several times a day.

As we move on to the last healing enhancer, a diet high in lysine, it is important to investigate how it can affect viral activity and aid in the healing of canker sores.

e. An important part of protein synthesis, immunological response, and viral suppression is the amino acid lysine. It is an important dietary supplement for the treatment of canker sores because of its capacity to suppress the activity of the herpes simplex virus (HSV), which is linked to the onset of these mouth ulcers. Through the consumption of foods high in lysine, people may be able to control the spread of viruses, lessen the intensity and duration of canker sores, and accelerate the healing process.

Studies have demonstrated how lysine affects viral activity, especially that of HSV, highlighting the supplement's potential to lessen the frequency and severity of mouth ulcers. In addition, people who have included a diet high in lysine in their regimen for managing canker sores have reported quicker healing and a lower incidence of oral ulcer recurrence.

People who want to relieve their canker sores may choose to include foods high in lysine in their diet, such as fish, eggs, dairy products, lentils, and lean meats. Furthermore, under the supervision of a medical practitioner, lysine supplements may be taken into consideration to guarantee sufficient consumption to promote the healing process of canker sores.

After a thorough investigation into healing boosters that might hasten the healing of canker sores, it is clear that an integrated strategy including these tactics can greatly improve the treatment and healing of these oral ulcers.

Finally, careful thought and application of healing enhancers like propolis extract, honey and turmeric paste, zinc supplementation, licorice paste, and a diet high in lysine can hasten the healing of canker sores, reduce discomfort associated with them, and encourage the restoration of dental health. Through an exploration of the intricate nuances of these restorative supplements and their real-world uses, people may equip themselves with comprehensive canker sore care techniques that will ultimately improve their well-being and quality of life.

As we move on to the next section of our investigation, we will continue to explore the complex strategy of managing canker sores in a comprehensive manner. We will also explore how oral hygiene practises, lifestyle changes, and other supportive strategies can be integrated to maximise oral health and well-being.

Preventive Measures at Home

As we go deeper into the preventive steps that may be taken at home to lessen the likelihood of these oral ulcers, we must continue our thorough investigation of total canker sore therapy. People can successfully lower their risk of getting canker sores by adopting these preventative practises on a regular basis, which will promote oral health and overall wellbeing. This chapter will explain a comprehensive list of preventive measures, each painstakingly explained to give a clear grasp of its workings, uses, and possible influence on the avoidance of canker sores.

A carefully compiled list of home remedies to help lessen the likelihood of developing canker sores is provided below:

Keeping your mouth as clean as possible is essential to avoiding canker sores. Using non-irritating oral care products in addition to regular brushing and flossing helps to get rid of bacteria and lower the risk of oral ulcers. Additionally, you can avoid oral tissue stress, which is frequently linked to the emergence of canker sores, by using a soft-bristled toothbrush and gentle brushing techniques.

Studies have repeatedly demonstrated the link between inadequate dental cleanliness and a higher risk of developing mouth ulcers, underscoring the importance of good oral hygiene in averting canker sores. In addition, people who follow strict oral hygiene guidelines report better dental health and a lower occurrence of canker sores.

People should emphasise maintaining a clean and healthy oral environment by using mouthwash without alcohol, flossing everyday, and brushing their teeth at least twice a day in order to prevent canker sores. Additionally, limiting oral tissue irritation can lower the likelihood of developing canker sores by choosing oral care products devoid of harsh chemicals and abrasives.

As we go on to the next preventive strategy, which is dietary adjustments, it is critical to investigate how nutritional decisions affect the avoidance of canker sores.

b. Canker sore prevention is greatly influenced by dietary variables. A balanced, diverse diet high in vital nutrients—iron, folate, and vitamin B12, in particular—can improve dental health and lower the risk of developing mouth ulcers. Canker sores can also be avoided by avoiding meals that are harsh and acidic since they can irritate the mouth mucosa.

Scientific literature has emphasised the impact of dietary practises and nutritional deficits on oral health, emphasising the function of particular nutrients in averting the development of canker sores. Oral ulcer incidence has also been reported to be lower among people who have adopted a well-balanced diet and minimised their consumption of possible irritants.

In order to prevent canker sores, people should make sure they are eating foods high in vitamin B12, including meat, fish, and dairy products, as well as foods high in iron and folate, like leafy greens, legumes, and fortified cereals. In addition, limiting the consumption of foods high in acidity, spice, and abrasiveness can protect the oral mucosa from irritation and help prevent canker sores.

Moving on to the next preventive strategy, which is stress management, it is important to examine the complex relationship that exists between dental health and psychological well-being.

d. One of the most important ways to stop canker sores from happening is to manage stress well. Oral ulcer susceptibility has been linked to chronic stress's thinning of the immune system and escalation of inflammatory processes. By using stress-reduction strategies like mindfulness, meditation, and relaxation exercises, one can lessen the negative effects of stress on dental health and lower the likelihood of getting canker sores.

Numerous studies have demonstrated the connection between psychological stress and oral health, highlighting the negative impacts of stress on immunological response and inflammatory processes in the mouth. Furthermore, people who have made stress management techniques a regular part of their lives have reported better general health and a reduction in the occurrence of canker sores.

People who want to prevent canker sores should prioritise stress management. They can do this by practising yoga, deep breathing techniques, and meditation, which reduce psychological tension and foster calm. In addition, preserving a good work-life balance and looking for social support will help lower stress levels generally, which will benefit oral health and stop canker sores from developing.

As we go on to the next preventive strategy, which is the avoidance of oral irritation, it is important to consider the importance of reducing potential irritants in order to stop the formation of canker sores.

d. Reducing oral irritation is essential to keeping canker sores at bay. By minimising oral mucosal stress and inflammation, smoking, abrasive toothpaste, and spicy foods, one can lessen the likelihood of getting oral ulcers. In addition, refraining from oral behaviours like tongue-cracking and cheek-biting can help avoid canker sores by preventing mechanical damage to the oral tissues.

The correlation between oral irritation and the occurrence of canker sores has been repeatedly observed in clinical observations and patient testimonies. This emphasises the significance of reducing potential irritants in order to prevent oral ulcers. Furthermore, people who have purposefully avoided oral irritants have reported better oral comfort and a reduction in the incidence of canker sores.

In order to prevent canker sores, people should use toothpaste that is gentler and less abrasive and steer clear of foods that are overly acidic or spicy as these can irritate the oral mucosa. In addition, the chance of developing canker sores can be effectively decreased by using stress-reduction strategies and being aware of one's oral habits in order to minimise unconscious oral tissue trauma.

As we move on to the last prophylactic, immune system support, it is relevant to investigate how immune function contributes to the avoidance of canker sores.

b. Preventing the development of canker sores requires immune system support. A balanced diet high in immune-boosting elements like zinc, vitamin D, and C, as well as adequate rest and exercise, helps strengthen the body's defences and lessen the risk of oral ulcers. Further supporting immune system function and encouraging good hygiene practises can help prevent canker sores by limiting exposure to infectious pathogens.

Numerous scientific studies have highlighted the importance of immune function for maintaining dental health and the effect that immune modulation has on preventing canker sores. Moreover, people who have made lifestyle changes that prioritise immune system support have reported better overall health and a lower frequency of oral ulcers.

People should make an effort to have a balanced lifestyle that includes enough sleep, frequent exercise, and a nutrient-dense diet rich in foods that strengthen the immune system, such as nuts, citrus fruits, and fatty fish, in order to support the immune system and avoid canker sores. At the same time, maintaining proper hygiene—which includes often washing your hands and limiting your exposure to potentially harmful substances—can strengthen your immune system and stop canker sores from developing.

A proactive attitude to oral health and well-being is crucial in preventing the development of these oral ulcers, as is made clear by the thorough investigation of preventive measures that may be used at home to lessen the incidence of canker sores.

In summary, the careful implementation of dental hygiene habits, dietary adjustments, stress reduction strategies, avoidance of oral irritation, and immune system stimulation can significantly lower the risk of getting canker sores, improving oral health and general wellbeing. Through a thorough examination of the intricate intricacies of these preventive measures and their real-world applications, people may equip themselves with comprehensive techniques for managing canker sores, which will eventually improve their quality of life.

As we move on to the next section of our investigation, we will continue to explore the complex strategy of managing canker sores in their entirety. We will also explore how to integrate professional care, lifestyle changes, and other supportive strategies to maximise oral health and overall wellbeing.

When Home Remedies Aren't Enough

After discussing the various preventive measures you may take at home to reduce your risk of getting a canker sore, let's discuss another crucial aspect of fully managing canker sores: knowing when to seek professional medical assistance. The expertise of medical specialists is sometimes required to treat and manage the complexities of canker sores, even while preventive measures and at-home therapies are crucial for maintaining oral health. This chapter will go into great detail on canker sore symptoms, potential treatments, and how to receive professional care. It will also cover the subtle indicators that should be taken seriously.

The primary issue at hand is how difficult it is to manage canker sores, especially knowing when it's crucial to seek professional medical assistance. Canker sores can create a lot of issues and discomfort, even though they are mostly benign. This can negatively impact a person's dental health and quality of life. However, in order to treat canker sores promptly and effectively, it is essential to recognise the signs and symptoms that point to the need for medical intervention.

Regarding canker sore treatment, failing to seek professional medical help when necessary can result in long-term pain, a worsening of the condition, and other challenges that may make it harder for the patient to go about their everyday lives and maintain good oral health. Ignoring the need for professional care can also lead to inadequate management of canker sores, which makes it more difficult to address the underlying issues that contribute to the sores' development and persistence.

To address this significant issue, it is required to elucidate the symptoms and circumstances that necessitate the involvement of medical professionals in the management of canker sores. By being aware of these symptoms, individuals can proactively seek expert guidance and care, which enhances the effectiveness of treating canker sores and promotes optimal oral health.

In order to detect the signs that necessitate seeking professional medical aid for the treatment of canker sores, it is crucial to comprehend the symptoms, their possible implications, and the best course of action to seek expert care. Using the expertise of healthcare professionals, managing the difficulties associated with canker sores requires a proactive approach to seeking professional advice and treatment.

Individuals who identify and act upon the indications of canker sores should anticipate improved symptom alleviation, increased oral comfort, and a proactive attitude towards addressing the underlying causes of these oral ulcers. Working together with healthcare experts, individuals can receive customised attention and tailored treatment programmes, leading to a more comprehensive and effective approach to managing canker sores.

While detecting symptoms that necessitate professional medical attention is crucial, it's also critical to acknowledge alternative choices that individuals may consider either in addition to or following professional medical attention. These may involve lifestyle modifications, adjuvant therapies, or additional supportive measures in addition to the professional management of canker sores in order to achieve total and holistic oral health.

After setting the framework, we look at the indications that indicate that canker sores require professional medical attention. We emphasise the critical role that medical professionals play in ensuring comprehensive and effective therapy.

a. Canker sores that require medical attention might present with a variety of symptoms and features that differ from how these oral ulcers usually progress. These consist of, but are not restricted to:

- Large or unusually shaped canker sores that cause significant discomfort and impair oral hygiene practises \s- Persistent or recurrent canker sores that significantly hinder daily activities and oral function \s- Canker sores accompanied by systemic symptoms like fever, malaise, or lymph node enlargement

- Canker sores developing with other oral lesions or worrisome oral alterations - Canker sores that, in spite of home cures and preventive measures, do not show any improvement or worsen over time

The significance of these unusual presentations has been highlighted by clinical observations and patient testimonies, highlighting the necessity of professional examination to identify underlying illnesses or contributory variables that may be aggravating the severity and duration of canker sores. Additionally, research has clarified the possible effects of these manifestations on a person's general dental health and well-being, highlighting the need for specialist care.

If someone experiences any of these unusual presentations, they should consult a dentist, an oral medicine expert, or a healthcare provider with an emphasis on oral pathology as soon as possible. In order to create a management strategy that is suited for each patient's unique needs and addresses the underlying causes of these unusual canker sore presentations, prompt assessment and diagnosis are essential.

b. A variety of examinations and inquiries are included in the diagnostic criteria that call for specialist care in the treatment of canker sores in order to determine the underlying cause, aggravating variables, and possible systemic effects of these mouth ulcers. These could consist of, but are not restricted to:

- Thorough oral examination to assess the features, location, and intensity of canker sores

- Cytologic analysis or biopsy of atypical or resistant canker sores to identify any possible dysplastic or neoplastic alterations

- Laboratory tests to determine whether nutritional deficits or underlying systemic problems are causing canker sore persistence.

- Imaging tests to look into deeper-seated oral lesions or related skeletal changes, such as oral radiography or sophisticated imaging modalities

- Specific diagnostic procedures to identify immune-mediated processes or other infection causes that could be causing canker sores

The importance of these diagnostic indicators is in their capacity to identify the underlying causes of unusual or persistent canker sores, hence assisting in the development of a suitable and focused treatment strategy. Additionally, patient testimonies have highlighted the importance of thorough diagnostic evaluations in clarifying the intricacies of the genesis and treatment of canker sores, highlighting the critical role that expert care plays in promoting successful outcomes.

People should aggressively seek out expert care from medical professionals when presented with these diagnostic indications. This will guarantee a comprehensive and customised diagnostic evaluation that will identify the underlying causes of atypical canker sore symptoms. Working together with medical professionals who specialise in oral pathology, oral medicine, or similar fields is crucial to developing a management plan that effectively tackles the unique causes and consequences of these mouth ulcers.

c. A wide range of treatment modalities and supportive measures are included in the therapeutic considerations and specific interventions for canker sores, with the goal of addressing the atypical symptoms and complexity of these oral ulcers. These could consist of, but are not restricted to:

- Targeted pharmaceutical treatments to reduce symptoms and encourage the cure of canker sores, such as corticosteroids, immunomodulators, or analgesics

- Topical therapies, such as corticosteroid preparations, gels, or specialty mouth rinses, can lessen discomfort and hasten the healing of unusual or chronic canker sores

- Adjunctive treatments to influence immune responses and encourage the healing of resistant canker sores, such as photobiomodulation, laser therapy, or other cutting-edge techniques.

- Referral to multidisciplinary medical professionals for the treatment of underlying systemic diseases or aggravating variables that prolong the course of canker sores

- Collaborative care, in which oral medicine experts, dentists, and other medical professionals create a thorough and customised treatment plan that meets each patient's unique needs

Through patient outcomes, expert consensus, and clinical studies, the effectiveness of various therapeutic considerations and specific therapies in controlling atypical or persistent canker sores has been established. Furthermore, patient narratives have emphasised the revolutionary influence of these customised treatment modalities in symptom relief, correcting atypical signs, and promoting oral comfort and well-being, underscoring their crucial function in specialised care.

After being diagnosed with a condition that requires specific care, patients should work closely with their healthcare professionals to develop and execute customised treatment plans and specialised management techniques. To create a thorough treatment plan that addresses the unique symptoms and underlying causes of unusual or persistent canker sores, this entails cooperative talks with oral medicine specialists, dentists, and other healthcare providers.

To sum up, in order to promote thorough and efficient care for canker sores, it is critical to recognise the warning symptoms that point to the need for professional medical intervention. People can more effectively manage canker sores and promote optimal dental health and well-being by proactively seeking professional examination and treatment when they recognise the unusual symptoms, diagnostic indicators, and therapeutic considerations that call for specialised care. Moving on to the next stage of our investigation, we will examine how to combine professional treatment, lifestyle adjustments, and other helpful techniques to maximise oral health and wellbeing—a comprehensive strategy that includes canker sore treatment.

Customizing Your Canker Sore Management Plan

Assessing Your Individual Triggers

This chapter's goal is to walk readers through the process of determining and successfully recording their own unique canker sore triggers. By the time this chapter ends, readers need to have a thorough grasp of the causes of their canker sore outbreaks and the resources necessary to control and lessen them.

Readers should have a fundamental awareness of canker sores, including their causes and symptoms, before starting the quest to identify specific triggers for canker sores. Throughout the process, it is also helpful to record observations and discoveries in a notebook or digital tool.

Evaluating personal causes of canker sores requires a multidisciplinary approach that takes into account a person's food, lifestyle, dental health, and general well-being. The first steps in the process are self-awareness and observation, which are then followed by methodical documentation and examination of possible triggers.

Readers can begin the process of pinpointing specific causes of canker sores by considering their daily schedules, eating patterns, and dental hygiene regimens. Any discernible trends or associations between particular actions or habits and the development of canker sores must be carefully considered. Furthermore, observing physical and mental stressors might provide important information about possible triggers.

Understanding the connection between dietary decisions and canker sore outbreaks is a crucial part of managing canker sores. It is recommended that readers keep a detailed journal of everything they eat and drink, including the kinds of foods and drinks they eat and how often they eat them. Readers who keep a thorough diet journal may be able to find links between specific foods and the development of canker sores.

Keeping your mouth clean is crucial to managing and avoiding canker sores. Readers should be particularly aware of their oral hygiene practises, including the kinds of mouthwash, toothpaste, and other products they use. Furthermore, it is imperative to document any modifications to dental hygiene protocols or the launch of novel products in order to evaluate their possible influence on the incidence of canker sores.

It is well known that stress can cause canker sores, thus its effects on dental health should not be undervalued. It is recommended that readers keep a check on their stress levels and recognise circumstances or occurrences that align with elevated stress. People can control their stress and lessen its impact on canker sore outbreaks by being aware of stressors and their impacts.

Hormonal fluctuations may be a factor in the development of canker sores, especially in women. Readers who identify as female should monitor their menstrual cycles and take note of any variations in the incidence of canker sores related to hormonal shifts. Comprehending the relationship between changes in hormone levels and canker sores is essential for a thorough evaluation of triggers. Consistency in recording observations and experiences is crucial during the trigger assessment procedure. Analytical data can be obtained by making thorough and consistent entries in a journal or digital instrument.

- It's critical to approach the process of finding triggers with an open mind and refrain from drawing hasty conclusions. It is important to confirm any correlations between specific causes and canker sore breakouts by regular observation and analysis.

- Without strong proof, readers should use caution when self-diagnosing triggers. Canker sores and certain circumstances have anecdotal relationships that need be verified by thorough recording and investigation.

Readers can examine the data to find patterns and possible triggers after compiling a sizable amount of information about their food habits, dental hygiene routines, stress levels, and hormone swings. Healthcare experts may be consulted as part of this investigation in order to confirm results and obtain new perspectives.

In the event that readers are unable to determine the specific factors that lead to canker sores, seeing dental health or dermatological specialists may be helpful. These experts can provide specific advice for trigger management as well as proficiency in recognising possible triggers.

In summary, identifying specific triggers for canker sores necessitates a methodical and thorough process that includes introspection, thorough recording, and critical analysis. Through meticulous monitoring of lifestyle variables, food consumption, dental hygiene habits, stress levels, and hormone shifts, readers can acquire important understanding of their individual triggers and equip themselves with the skills necessary to control and lessen canker sore outbreaks. This proactive strategy to stimulate assessment and self-awareness set the stage for better oral health and effective management of canker sores.

Creating a Tailored Diet Plan

This chapter's goal is to give readers a foundation for creating a diet plan that takes into account their unique dietary triggers and nutritional requirements. Readers should be able to design a customised diet plan targeted at controlling and avoiding canker sores by the end of this chapter, having gained a thorough grasp of how dietary decisions can influence canker sore breakouts.

As mentioned in the last chapter, readers should have finished assessing their personal triggers for canker sores before diving into the process of designing a customised nutrition plan. To properly put this chapter's advice into practise, it also helps to have a basic awareness of nutrition and dietary principles.

Creating a customised diet plan for the treatment of canker sores requires a comprehensive strategy that takes into account the interactions between dietary triggers, dietary needs, and general health. The procedure includes determining which nutrients are helpful, assessing possible food triggers, and creating a sustainable, well-balanced diet plan that suits each person's needs and tastes.

Finding Possible Food Allergens

Expanding on the knowledge acquired from the evaluation of certain triggers, readers ought to go over their recorded observations about food consumption and canker sore incidences. Through the examination of trends and relationships between particular foods, drinks, or eating behaviours and the development of canker sores, readers can pinpoint dietary triggers that might be responsible for their oral health issues. Citrus fruits, nuts, food additives, and acidic or spicy foods are examples of common triggers.

Meeting with a Nutritionist or Registered Dietitian for Advice

Getting advice from a certified nutritionist can be very helpful in developing a customised dietary plan for the treatment of canker sores. A qualified nutritionist or registered dietitian can assist people in evaluating their eating patterns, locating possible trigger foods, and creating a customised nutrition plan that fits their unique requirements and supports their overall health objectives. Getting professional advice can help with nutritional shortages, make the best dietary choices, and guarantee a sustainable and well-balanced approach to managing canker sores.

Stressing the Use of Nutrient-Rich Foods

To maintain dental health and lower the risk of canker sore outbreaks, a diet rich in nutrient-dense foods must be included. The consumption of foods high in vitamins, especially vitamin B12, vitamin C, and folate, should be prioritised by readers because these nutrients are essential for maintaining the health of the oral mucosa. Probiotics, iron, and zinc supplements can also support immune system and dental health in general, which may lessen the incidence and severity of canker sores.

Avoiding or Moderating Trigger Foods

Readers should make educated judgments about including, limiting, or avoiding particular foods and beverages that are known to worsen symptoms of canker sores based on the identified dietary triggers. Readers are advised to use caution when consuming acidic, spicy, or abrasive foods and to keep an eye on their mouth reactions to these dietary choices, even if individual tolerance to trigger foods may vary. People can reduce the possible impact on the occurrence of canker sores and proactively manage their food triggers by implementing thoughtful and planned dietary alterations.

Customizing the Diet Plan

In order to create a customised diet plan that meets their unique requirements, readers should seek professional help while considering their own tastes, dietary restrictions, and nutritional requirements. This diet should include a wide variety of foods high in nutrients, a balanced consumption of macronutrients, and thoughtful adjustments to address trigger foods that have been identified. The food plan should also be flexible and durable so that canker sore triggers can be managed over the long run and long-term adherence is possible.

- Maintaining a balanced and diverse diet is crucial when applying dietary alterations to control triggers for canker sores in order to ensure proper nutrient intake and general health.

- Restrictive dietary methods should be avoided by readers as they may result in imbalances or deficits in certain nutrients. A trained expert can guide people through dietary changes while ensuring that their nutritional needs are met.

- Dietary adjustments should be made with care and patience because it may take some time and regular observation to see how they affect the incidence of canker sores. Changes in diet that are sudden or significant should be made carefully and under the advice of a professional.

After developing a customised diet plan, readers can assess its efficacy by tracking the frequency and intensity of canker sore outbreaks in connection to dietary changes. Maintaining thorough documentation of food consumption and canker sore incidences can help identify important feedback regarding the effectiveness of the diet plan and guide future improvements.

In the event that readers experience difficulties carrying out or sticking to their customised diet plan, consulting a qualified dietitian or nutritionist on a regular basis might provide answers to frequent problems. Expert advice can help with managing dietary issues, fine-tuning the diet, and overcoming any obstacles pertaining to dietary changes and canker sore care.

In summary, developing a customised diet plan for the treatment of canker sores requires a methodical and individualised strategy that incorporates knowledge from nutritional assessments, trigger assessments, and personal dietary preferences. Through a customised sustainable diet plan, identification of potential trigger foods, and an emphasis on nutrient-rich options, readers can take charge of their health and prevent canker sores by managing their diet in a proactive manner. This comprehensive and knowledgeable approach to nutrition management establishes the groundwork for better oral health and overall wellbeing.

Selecting the Right Supplements

Canker sore treatment goes beyond dietary changes to include a multifaceted strategy that combines several approaches to target specific triggers and maintain dental health. Taking into account appropriate supplements based on a person's health profile and canker sore patterns becomes important when trying to control canker sores effectively. People might potentially address specific deficiencies, improve oral mucosal health, and lessen the frequency and severity of canker sore breakouts by adding targeted nutrients and chemicals to their diet.

Notwithstanding the possible advantages of supplementation in the treatment of canker sores, people may find it difficult to choose the proper supplements that suit their individual demands and health profile. Supplementation cannot be effectively integrated into a holistic management approach if there is a lack of tailored counsel and an overwhelming assortment of supplements accessible. This might cause confusion and doubt.

Individuals may suffer from persistent nutritional deficits, reduced oral mucosal integrity, and increased vulnerability to canker sore outbreaks if they do not take supplements that are appropriate for their specific health profiles and canker sore patterns. Inadequate supplementation may have negative effects on overall health and quality of life, including longer discomfort, delayed healing, and an increased burden of maintaining recurrent canker sores.

The problem of choosing the best supplements for the treatment of canker sores requires a systematic strategy that combines expert advice, evidence-based selection criteria, and customised assessment. People can maximise the potential advantages of supplementation in promoting oral health and reducing the burden of canker sores by navigating the varied terrain of supplements with a personalised focus on individual health needs and canker sore patterns.

There are a number of important phases involved in choosing the best supplements for managing canker sores, and each one helps to ensure that supplementing is individualised and well-informed when it comes to a patient's overall management plan.

Personalized Health Assessment

The cornerstone for choosing the right supplements is a thorough evaluation of each person's health status, including nutritional deficits, dental health indicators, and underlying disorders. People can learn more about their unique health needs and possible areas for targeted supplementing by consulting with healthcare specialists, such as a dentist or primary care physician.

Identification of Targeted Nutrients and Compounds

Expanding on the customised health evaluation, it is critical to identify specific nutrients and chemicals relevant to the management of canker sores. Important factors might include the functions of vitamins, minerals, and bioactive substances in promoting immune system modulation, addressing potential canker sore triggers, and maintaining the health of the oral mucosa. Supplementation decisions can be made to best maximise the possible influence on management strategy by matching individual demands and canker sore patterns.

Evidence-Based Selection Criteria

Using evidence-based selection criteria can help you make sense of the wide range of supplements that are out there. Supplements with scientific data backing them up should be given priority by people who want to treat oral health issues, manage canker sore causes, and improve their general well-being. With the help of this evidence-based methodology, people are better equipped to make knowledgeable judgments about which supplements to take and may base their selections on verified advantages and possible results.

Professional Guidance and Collaboration

Selecting supplements is made much easier by consulting with knowledgeable healthcare providers, such as a pharmacist, registered dietitian, or other healthcare professional with experience in nutritional supplementation. Working with experts allows people to get tailored advice, understand possible drug interactions with current diseases or drugs, and maximise how well-suited certain supplements are for their overall health care.

A tailored approach to choosing the best supplements for managing canker sores has the potential to yield great results and enhance oral health and overall well-being. Through the use of evidence-based selection criteria, individual health needs, and expert assistance, people can expect better management of their overall health profile, decreased incidence of canker sores, and increased support for oral mucosal integrity.

Although dietary changes and supplements are frequently the mainstay of canker sore care, other approaches including topical therapies, stress reduction methods, and good dental hygiene habits may also be beneficial to the all-encompassing approach. People ought to think about integrating many methods in a comprehensive way that is specific to their canker sore patterns and needs. This can improve the efficacy of their management efforts in a cooperative manner.

To sum up, choosing the appropriate supplements based on a person's health history and canker sore patterns is an essential part of an all-encompassing treatment plan. By using a systematic, individualised approach that includes health assessment, evidence-based selection criteria, and professional collaboration, people can make sense of the supplement landscape and maximise its potential benefits in maintaining oral health and lessening the effects of canker sores. This well-informed and customised supplement integration supports a proactive, all-encompassing approach to managing canker sores, which in turn promotes better oral health and general wellbeing.

Integrating Holistic Practices Into Daily Life

Our intention in this area is to inspire readers to incorporate holistic practises into their daily lives in order to prevent canker sores and to promote general well-being. We hope to enable readers to take charge of their dental health and lessen the impact of canker sore outbreaks by offering a road map for implementing holistic treatments.

It takes a commitment to prioritising self-care and a readiness to embrace lifestyle adjustments to incorporate holistic practises into daily life. Although there are no required resources, readers should be willing to investigate different holistic therapies and commit the necessary time and energy to incorporating these practises into their daily routine.

The amalgamation of holistic practises comprises a diverse approach that includes dietary modifications, stress mitigation strategies, dental hygiene regimens, and mindfulness exercises. People who embrace a holistic approach can foster an atmosphere that promotes dental health and general well-being, which lays the groundwork for preventing canker sores.

Dietary Modifications

Starting with dietary changes, people can maximise their intake to promote dental health and reduce the incidence of canker sores. The promotion of immune function and oral mucosal integrity can be achieved by incorporating nutrient-dense foods such as fruits, vegetables, lean meats, and whole grains into a well-rounded diet. Including anti-inflammatory foods like ginger, turmeric, and omega-3 fatty acids can also aid in the management of canker sores and lessen oral irritation.

Stress Management Techniques

Understanding how stress affects dental health, people can reduce possible causes of canker sores by implementing stress-reduction strategies into their daily lives. Exercises that promote emotional balance and mindfulness, including as yoga, meditation, and deep breathing, can help maintain oral mucosal health and lessen the effects of stress-related canker sore outbreaks.

Oral Hygiene Practices

An essential component of comprehensive oral care is placing a high priority on oral cleanliness. By following consistent brushing and flossing protocols, using mouthwashes that include natural antiseptic qualities, and staying well-hydrated, people can foster an environment that promotes oral health and lessens the risk of developing canker sores. Additionally, maintaining the integrity of the oral mucosa and preventing canker sores is facilitated by avoiding abrasive dental products and practising gentle oral hygiene.

Mindfulness Activities

Including mindfulness exercises like journaling, gratitude exercises, and self-analysis promotes resilience and emotional well-being, which in turn promotes general health and the management of canker sores. People can improve their capacity to manage stress and adjust to possible triggers by developing a positive outlook and developing self-awareness, which will ultimately promote a comprehensive approach to oral health and well-being.

- Tips:
- Introduce dietary changes gradually to allow for adaptation and adjustment.

Try out various stress-reduction strategies to find the ones that work best for your requirements.

- To reduce the chance of causing canker sores, choose dental care products that are free of any irritants and allergies.

Adopt a customised approach to mindfulness exercises, customising methods to suit particular tastes and way of life.

- Warnings: - Avoid making abrupt or significant dietary changes as these can affect dental health and upset digestive systems.

- When choosing stress-reduction strategies, practise mindfulness and make sure the methods you choose fit your comfort level and skill level.

- To avoid unfavourable responses and oral irritations, be aware of any allergies or sensitivities in oral care products.

In order to verify the effective incorporation of holistic practises into everyday life, people should keep an eye on their oral health and well-being, noting any changes in the frequency of canker sores, their stress levels, and their general resilience. Furthermore, getting input from medical specialists like dentists or holistic practitioners can shed light on how holistic approaches affect dental health and the treatment of canker sores.

If there are difficulties or obstacles in incorporating holistic approaches, people should reevaluate their strategy, consult with medical professionals, and think about modifying their tactics to fit their unique requirements and situation. In order to overcome any roadblocks and improve the incorporation of holistic practises into everyday life, flexibility and adaptation are crucial.

To sum up, incorporating holistic practises into daily life is an empowering and proactive way to support general well-being and prevent canker sores. People can foster resistance against potential triggers for canker sores and establish a supportive environment for oral health by adopting dietary changes, stress management strategies, oral hygiene routines, and mindfulness exercises. By adopting a committed and all-encompassing strategy, individuals can utilise these techniques to improve their dental health and overall wellbeing, thereby adding to the entire guide for managing canker sores.

Designing a Stress Management Program

This section's goal is to assist readers in creating a customised stress management plan that fits their needs, interests, and stressors. We hope to enable people to proactively address and lessen the negative effects of stress on their general well-being by providing a methodical approach.

Creating a stress management programme requires being open-minded, prepared to try out different stress-reduction strategies, and determined to put self-care first. While there are no required supplies, readers should be ready to put in some time and effort to put the program's strategies into practise.

Identifying stressors, researching stress management strategies, creating a customised stress management plan, and incorporating stress-relieving activities into everyday life are all steps in the process of creating a stress management programme. People can develop resilience and improve their capacity to manage stress by implementing these strategies.

Identifying Stressors

Finding the precise stressors that have an effect on a person's well-being is the first step in creating a stress management programme. Through introspection, identification of stressors, and evaluation of the sources of stress, people can learn more about the elements that influence their stress levels. The basis for creating focused stress management techniques is this self-awareness.

Exploring Stress Management Techniques

Once stressors have been identified, people can investigate a variety of stress-reduction strategies to determine which ones work best for them. Practices including progressive muscular relaxation, yoga, tai chi, deep breathing techniques, and mindfulness meditation may fall under this category. People can find the methods that best suit their interests and resonate with them by experimenting with these tactics.

Developing a Personalized Stress Management Plan

People can create a customised stress management strategy by using the knowledge they obtain from recognising stressors and researching stress management strategies. This plan ought to include a comprehensive range of techniques designed to deal with particular stressors and advance general wellbeing. To effectively manage stress, a mix of cognitive, emotional, and physical strategies may be used.

Integrating Stress-Relief Practices into Daily Life

Integrating the customised stress management strategy into day-to-day activities is the last phase in this approach. This could be scheduling specific time for stress-relieving activities, including mindfulness into regular activities, creating boundaries to reduce stressors, and creating a welcoming environment that supports stress management. Integrating these principles into one's lifestyle requires dedication and consistency.

- Tips:

- To encourage gradual adaption, start with tiny, doable modifications when using stress management approaches.

Try out a range of stress-relieving techniques before deciding on a customised stress-reduction strategy.

Stress self-compassion and patience as essential qualities during the planning and execution of a stress management programme.

- Tailor the stress management strategy to each person's values, inclinations, and daily schedule.

- Caution: - Avoid using excessively strict or unrealistic stress management techniques as they may exacerbate existing tension or frustration.

- Refrain from comparing your own development to that of others, since every person's journey towards stress management is distinct and intimate.

- When incorporating stress-relieving techniques into your everyday life, consider balance and be aware of the possibility of burnout from overcommitting to these techniques.

In order to verify the efficacy of the stress management programme, people should keep an eye on their stress levels, emotional stability, and general resilience. Feedback on the effectiveness of the stress management techniques that have been put into practise can be obtained by monitoring shifts in stress reactions and individual coping techniques. Consulting peers or mental health professionals might provide further insights into the efficacy of the customised stress management approach.

If there are problems or obstacles in putting the stress management programme into practise, people are urged to review their strategy, get help from mental health specialists, and modify their tactics to better suit their changing needs. In order to maximise the influence of the customised stress management plan on overall well-being, flexibility and adaptation are essential.

In summary, the process of creating a customised stress management programme gives people the skills and knowledge they need to deal with stress and foster resilience. Readers can create a proactive approach to stress management and overall well-being by identifying stressors, investigating stress-relief approaches, creating a tailored stress management plan, and incorporating these practises into daily life.

Monitoring and Adapting Your Plan

When it comes to canker sore care, it is important to understand that a number of factors, including individual variances in response to medications, lifestyle modifications, and the possibility of recurrence, can affect how well the management plan works. As a result, keeping an eye on the treatment plan's development and making the required adjustments are crucial to the ongoing effectiveness of reducing pain and the interference that canker sores cause with daily activities.

The main problem at hand is that the canker sore management plan needs to be monitored and adjusted more proactively. In the absence of this preventive measure, people can endure protracted discomfort, a rise in the frequency of canker sore eruptions, and difficulties with day-to-day functions including speaking, eating, and brushing their teeth.

People with canker sores may have extended periods of discomfort, increased anxiety or stress associated with canker sore outbreaks, and possible interruptions to their oral health and general well-being if the management plan is not routinely reviewed and modified. In addition, therapies may be less successful and patients may feel helpless or frustrated about adequately controlling canker sores if the management plan is not modified.

Given the dynamic nature of canker sores, a thorough approach to monitoring and modifying the care plan is necessary. People can make educated judgments about changing their management plan to better fit their changing needs by putting in place a systematic framework for monitoring treatment efficacy and detecting possible triggers.

There are several important phases in putting the solution into practise. First and foremost, people ought to maintain a thorough log of all of their canker sore events, including the frequency, length, and intensity of outbreaks. In order to make continued tracking and analysis easier, this record can be kept in a spreadsheet, digital app, or notebook. People should also record any dietary, lifestyle, stress, and dental hygiene changes that may have an effect on the development of canker sores. This thorough documentation will provide as a basis for assessing the present management plan's efficacy and pinpointing possible areas for change.

In addition, frequent meetings with oral health specialists or dentists can yield insightful information about how the management plan is doing as well as professional suggestions for improvements. These specialists are able to perform comprehensive evaluations of oral health, offer customised treatment plans, and assist patients in fine-tuning their management strategy in light of the particulars of their canker sores and general state of oral health.

Positive outcomes, such as a decrease in the frequency and severity of canker sore outbreaks, enhanced coping strategies for managing discomfort, and an increased sense of control over the impact of canker sores on daily life, are expected from the systematic monitoring and modification of the management plan. By means of meticulous monitoring and deliberate adjustments to the treatment strategy, people can maximise their method of managing canker sores and enjoy improved comfort and oral health.

The suggested strategy places a strong emphasis on methodical monitoring and plan adaption, but it's important to recognise that there are other options that could improve or supplement the management of canker sores. These could involve changing one's diet to eliminate possible trigger foods, practising stress-reduction strategies like mindfulness meditation or relaxation techniques, and thinking about supplementary therapy like dental hygiene products or topical treatments designed to relieve canker sores. To make sure that these alternate solutions are compatible with each person's needs and preferences, evaluation of them should be informed by evidence-based research and individualised considerations.

To summarise, the proactive monitoring and modification of the canker sore management plan are essential for maximising canker sore treatment and reducing the impact on everyday activities. Through methodical monitoring of treatment outcomes, consulting with experts, and making educated adjustments based on personal experiences, people can take charge of their canker sore treatment process and promote enhanced oral comfort and overall well-being.

When to Seek Professional Help

One of the most important aspects of comprehensive care for canker sores is the idea of getting professional assistance. Aphthous ulcers, another name for canker sores, can range in severity and may require medical competence to guarantee proper diagnosis, treatment, and continued support. For people navigating the complexity of canker sore management, it is imperative that they recognise the signs that point to the need for expert assistance and know how to get it.

Seeking professional assistance is the proactive engagement of medical professionals for the assessment, diagnosis, and treatment of canker sores, such as dentists, oral health specialists, or physicians. This involvement could take several forms, such as getting expert insight into the underlying causes of canker sores, getting recommendations for specific treatments, and getting access to specialised care for severe or recurrent episodes.

Choosing to consult a doctor for canker sores entails a number of important factors. In order to handle the complex nature of canker sores, it first requires realising the limitations of self-management techniques and the potential advantages of professional competence. Seeking expert assistance also means taking an active role in the diagnosis process, which could include talking about medical history, doing extensive oral examinations, and possibly conducting more tests to determine the underlying causes of canker sore development.

Furthermore, getting professional assistance for canker sores includes creating individualised treatment plans that are catered to each patient's unique requirements and situation. This could entail prescribing specific drugs, offering complementary treatments, or putting preventive measures in place with the goal of reducing the severity and likelihood of canker sore recurrence.

Even though the historical or etymological background of getting professional assistance for canker sores may not be as well-known as it is in other fields, it is important to acknowledge how oral healthcare is changing and how individualised, evidence-based treatments for oral conditions are becoming more and more important. The advancement of dentistry and oral health practises throughout history has aided in the creation of novel treatment modalities, the integration of interdisciplinary approaches to treat oral mucosal problems, such as canker sores, and the improvement of diagnostic techniques.

It is important to place the idea of getting expert assistance for canker sores within the larger context of complete oral healthcare. This involves realising the need of collaborative care involving multiple healthcare providers, the relationship between oral health and systemic well-being, and the critical role that patient education and empowerment play in delivering the best possible oral health outcomes. By placing the act of requesting professional assistance within this broad framework, people are better able to understand the interrelated aspects of managing canker sores and the potential benefits of interdisciplinary cooperation.

Examples of situations in which people seek professional assistance for canker sores in real life include those in which they suffer from recurrent or exceptionally severe bouts of canker sores that have a major negative influence on their quality of life. When people seek professional help, they can decrease the burden of canker sores on their daily activities and improve their coping mechanisms by receiving precise diagnoses, focused treatment approaches, and continuous support. Furthermore, real-world applications include situations in which patients may need specialist care to manage canker sores in the context of underlying systemic conditions, such as immune-mediated diseases or dietary deficiencies, requiring the knowledge and skills of medical professionals with specific training in these fields.

The idea that getting expert assistance for canker sores is only necessary in cases that are severe or persistent is a prevalent fallacy. It is vital to refute this misunderstanding and underscore that obtaining expert aid is advantageous for all types of canker sore encounters, even the mildest ones. People can take proactive measures to address potential triggers, receive individualised recommendations, and form a collaborative partnership focused at enhancing their dental health and well-being by interacting with healthcare practitioners early in the course of managing canker sores.

In summary, the notion of obtaining expert assistance for the treatment of canker sores entails a complex strategy that combines therapeutic, diagnostic, and supporting components to meet the various needs of those impacted by these lesions of the oral mucosa. People can treat canker sores more effectively by adopting the proactive involvement of healthcare professionals. This will provide them with improved knowledge, individualised interventions, and a greater sense of empowerment to maximise their oral health and general well-being.

Navigating Social Situations

Dining Out With Dietary Restrictions

For those who have dietary restrictions, eating out can be difficult because there are frequently fewer options and a risk of coming into contact with allergens or irritants. In today's world, when more individuals are becoming aware of food allergies and intolerances and adopting specialised diets for moral or health-related reasons, this topic is very important.

The main problem here is how hard it is for those with certain dietary needs to eat out. This involves the possibility of eating something that contains allergies, the scarcity of appropriate menu options, and the possibility of feeling left out of social dining occasions.

For people with dietary restrictions, ignoring this issue may have a number of detrimental effects. These could include negative health outcomes from allergy exposure, depressive and lonely sentiments, and a dislike of eating out, which can affect social interactions and mental health.

People with dietary restrictions can use a variety of techniques to successfully navigate restaurant menus and communicate their needs to service members in order to overcome these problems. They can minimise the hazards related to their dietary restrictions and improve their eating experiences by doing this.

It's important to study restaurants that can accommodate particular dietary demands in advance when dining out with dietary restrictions. This could entail looking through internet menus, making advance contact with the eatery, or getting referrals from people who have experienced similar things. It's also critical to let restaurant employees know about any dietary restrictions and any allergies. This can be accomplished by asking pertinent questions on menu items and food preparation techniques, as well as by gently but firmly expressing specific needs.

People who have dietary requirements should take the initiative to speak out for what they need in order to guarantee a secure and pleasurable dining experience. Furthermore, knowing common allergens and hidden components as well as having a thorough awareness of one's dietary restrictions can help one make educated decisions while choosing dishes from the menu.

Individuals with dietary restrictions can greatly enhance their dining-out experiences by putting these suggestions into practise. When navigating restaurant menus, they are probably going to feel more empowered and competent, which will increase their sense of inclusion and enjoyment during social dining events. Furthermore, people can lessen the possibility of allergy exposure and the possible drawbacks of eating out while adhering to dietary restrictions by clearly explaining their demands to restaurant workers.

Even though the previously mentioned tactics work well, it's important to think of other approaches to deal with the difficulties of eating out while adhering to dietary restrictions. To guarantee a secure and comfortable dining atmosphere, some people might decide to cook at home and organise social gatherings, while others might prefer to dine at restaurants that specialise in meeting particular dietary needs. But these options might not always be available or preferred, which is why the above-mentioned tactics are especially helpful for people who want to enjoy eating out but still keep their dietary limitations under control.

In conclusion, many people find that eating out while adhering to dietary restrictions is a major difficulty; nevertheless, these difficulties can be lessened with proper preparation and good communication. People with dietary restrictions can prioritise their health and well-being while enjoying good dining experiences by using the techniques described in this chapter to communicate their needs to restaurant personnel, confidently explore restaurant menus, and prioritise their dining experiences. Individuals who have dietary restrictions can fully participate in the culinary pleasures that enhance our lives and thrive in social dining settings if they take a proactive approach and are ready to advocate for their requirements.

Explaining Canker Sores to Others

Fostering empathy and support for those who suffer with canker sores requires educating friends, family, and coworkers on the nature of the ailment. Phthous ulcers, another name for canker sores, are painful, recurring lesions that appear on the palate, inner cheeks, gums, tongue, and soft tissues inside the mouth. They can have a major effect on a person's quality of life by influencing their ability to speak, eat, and feel comfortable in general. To promote understanding, support, and productive communication, it is crucial to arm others in the vicinity of people suffering from canker sores with thorough knowledge.

The main problem is that the general public is unaware of and misinformed about the incapacitating consequences of canker sores. Unaware of the severe suffering and disturbance they can bring to the lives of those afflicted, many people view canker sores as mere annoyances. This ignorance could result in misunderstandings and hurtful comments, which would increase the emotional strain on those who have canker sores.

If this lack of knowledge is not addressed, people who have canker sores may feel alone, misinterpreted, and unsupported. Managing recurrent canker sores can have a significant emotional cost, resulting in stress, anxiety, and a decreased quality of life. Furthermore, people may suffer longer if they are unaware of the causes and treatments for canker sores, which may prevent them from getting the proper medical attention and from taking preventative action.

Establishing transparent and educational avenues to explain the nature of canker sores and their effects on people is crucial to closing this knowledge gap. By eliminating myths and offering correct information, the general public can create a more understanding and encouraging atmosphere for people who are coping with canker sores. In the end, this may lessen the stigma attached to this illness by raising awareness and understanding.

The successful application of this approach depends on friends, family, and coworkers being informed about canker sores in a clear and accurate manner. Open dialogues, instructional materials, and internet resources that describe the causes, symptoms, and treatment options for canker sores can all help achieve this. Role-playing exercises and empathy-building techniques can also be used to assist people comprehend the difficulties faced by those who have canker sores.

People with canker sores are likely to receive more understanding and support from their social circles if they educate others on the intricacies of the ailment and its effects. This may result in enhanced mental health and a setting that is better suited for handling and overcoming canker sores. Additionally, people may seek early intervention and take preventive action if they are more aware of the triggers and management strategies for canker sores. This might potentially lessen the frequency and severity of their episodes.

Although the suggested remedy places a strong emphasis on awareness-raising and education, other strategies might entail starting online forums or support groups where people who have canker sores can exchange stories and knowledge. These online communities may be extremely helpful for those who have canker sores as well as the people who care about them. They provide a supportive community as well as a plethora of useful tips and coping mechanisms. Furthermore, increasing public awareness through media campaigns and neighbourhood gatherings can advance a culture of empathy and support and foster a deeper knowledge of canker sores.

To sum up, helping others understand, empathise with, and provide support for those who suffer with this chronic and sometimes misdiagnosed ailment is crucial. We can foster a more welcoming and encouraging atmosphere that enables people with canker sores to successfully manage their illness and lead satisfying lives by practising open communication and education.

Social Eating Strategies

This section's main goal is to give people who have canker sores practical advice on how to handle social eating situations without making their symptoms worse. With the help of this thorough guide on handling meals in social situations, readers will acquire the self-assurance and understanding required to reduce discomfort and relish eating occasions without needless worry or suffering.

It is crucial for readers to comprehend their unique canker sore triggers and management strategies before starting the road of mastering social eating practises, as explained in the preceding chapters. Access to appropriate oral care products, like numbing gels and gentle mouthwashes, may also be helpful in putting the ideas mentioned into practise.

Learning how to use social eating methods entails a number of essential skills, such as meal planning in advance, choosing appropriate foods and drinks, navigating dining etiquette, and controlling discomfort during and after meals. All of these elements play a part in achieving the ultimate objective of providing people with canker sores with a pleasant and cosy dining experience.

1. Those with canker sores should think about looking over the menu or talking with the host or restaurant personnel about their food options before attending a social event or eating occasion. This proactive strategy can assist in identifying appropriate meal selections and possible trigger items to stay away from.

2. Choosing mild, non-spicy, and non-acidic foods will help reduce canker sore aggravation. Furthermore, avoiding discomfort can be achieved by selecting cold or lukewarm drinks over hot or fizzy ones.

3.: A more comfortable eating experience can be achieved by discreetly discussing dietary requirements or preferences with the host or service. It is imperative to manage this correspondence with grace and elegance in order to prevent undue attention being paid to one's condition.

4.:- If soreness from a canker sore appears during or after a meal, having oral care supplies on hand, such as light mouthwashes or numbing gels, can offer convenient relief while travelling. Eating slowly and with caution might help lessen the chance of escalating pre-existing sores.

Prioritize simple or bland dishes like steamed veggies, rice, or mild soups when perusing the menu because they are less likely to cause discomfort from canker sores.

-: Foods that are hot, spicy, acidic, crunchy, or difficult to chew should be avoided since they may present difficulties for people who have canker sores.

Talking to others and interacting socially while eating can help take the attention off of any discomfort and make eating more pleasurable.

Following the implementation of these tactics, people can evaluate their eating experiences in order to ascertain the efficacy of the recommended approaches. This could entail evaluating the degree of discomfort felt, the effectiveness of prior planning, and the general enjoyment of social dining occasions.

If during a social meal there is sudden discomfort or worsening of the symptoms of a canker sore, people can quietly leave the meal to take care of the problem, using oral care items if they are accessible. Furthermore, during difficult dining situations, support and understanding can be given by a valued confidant or partner who is aware of one's condition.

To sum up, developing social eating skills is an essential part of managing canker sores since it helps people to eat and socialise with confidence and little discomfort. Notwithstanding the difficulties caused by canker sores, people can develop a more positive and pleasurable relationship with food and social interactions by adhering to the comprehensive instructions offered in this part and putting the advice into practise.

Networking and Professional Settings

People who have canker sores in the workplace frequently encounter particular difficulties when interacting in professional settings and networking activities. Canker sores can be uncomfortable and distracting, which might affect a person's confidence and capacity to connect professionally. Therefore, it is essential to discuss canker sore management in professional settings so that people can stay composed and concentrate on their work goals.

The principal concern that needs to be addressed is the possible obstacle that canker sores provide in work settings. Painful mouth ulcers known as canker sores can be uncomfortable, make it harder to talk, and make you feel more self-conscious. These symptoms may make it difficult for people to network and communicate successfully in work environments, which may have an impact on their professional reputation and chances for career progression.

Untreated canker sores can have a variety of negative effects on a person, such as diminished self-esteem, the possibility that clients or coworkers will misinterpret their discomfort, and a weakened capacity to communicate knowledge and professionalism. Furthermore, the discomfort and diversion brought on by canker sores could make them less focused on forming valuable business connections and taking advantage of networking opportunities.

People can take a proactive stance that includes both preventive steps and discomfort management techniques to get over the difficulties in dealing with canker sores in work environments. Through the implementation of focused solutions, individuals can reduce the negative effects of canker sores on their professional relationships and confidently and easily maintain their professional appearance.

The management of canker sores in work environments requires a multimodal strategy that includes preventative actions as well as mobile management techniques. To guarantee that one's condition does not interfere with professional relationships, this entails knowing one's own triggers, organising professional activities in advance, discretely managing discomfort, and communicating effectively.

By using these treatments, people can anticipate increased confidence, increased comfort, and an increased capacity to concentrate on work-related activities without being distracted by discomfort from canker sores. People can handle professional environments with professionalism and poise by taking proactive care of their condition and using effective techniques. This will maximise their networking opportunities and prospects for career growth.

Even though the suggested remedies provide a thorough method for handling canker sores in work environments, it's crucial to recognise that every person is different and has different wants and preferences. Examining substitute approaches, like dietary adjustments, stress reduction methods, or different dental care items, might offer people more ways to deal with their particular problems in work settings.

Canker sore care goes beyond treating physical pain when it comes to social gatherings and work environments. It touches on important facets of self-presentation, self-assurance, and effective communication. In order to equip people to handle networking events and professional contacts with professionalism and confidence, the following sections will explore the specific tactics and workable solutions for managing canker sores in professional settings.

Romantic Relationships and Intimacy

Intimacy maintenance and expectation management are essential for creating a happy and healthy partnership in love relationships. Relationship dynamics can be complicated, and people frequently struggle to maintain closeness and deal with the range of expectations that come with being in a partnership. In order to make sure that romantic relationships flourish and last throughout time, these factors must be taken care of.

The main problem in romantic relationships is the mismatch in expectations between partners and the possible deterioration of intimacy. Emotional, physical, and psychological closeness are all parts of intimacy, and when these ties break down, it can cause feelings of alienation and discontent. Moreover, friction and tension resulting from different expectations between partners can negatively affect the harmony of the partnership as a whole.

There may be serious repercussions if the issues surrounding intimacy and expectations in romantic relationships are not resolved. Feelings of emotional distance, loneliness, and a drop in overall relationship satisfaction can result from a lack of intimacy. Furthermore, unfulfilled expectations can lead to friction, broken communication, and anger inside the partnership, which can cause relationship discomfort or even breakup.

Couples can take proactive measures to foster closeness and skillfully manage expectations in order to address these issues. To achieve this, prioritise spending quality time with each other, foster open and honest communication, and make an effort to comprehend and match each other's expectations for the relationship. Couples can create a stronger link and a deeper feeling of understanding by putting these strategies into practise.

It takes intentional work and dedication from both partners to put ideas for preserving intimacy and controlling expectations in love relationships into practise. This entails having frequent, meaningful discussions about one another's wants and goals, participating in intimate and understanding-fostering activities, and making a concerted effort to actively and respectfully satisfy one another's expectations.

Couples can anticipate increased communication, deeper connection, and better expectation alignment in their relationship when these solutions are put into practise. Couples can cultivate a more harmonious and satisfying partnership and increase the duration and general contentment of their relationship by giving priority to these characteristics and making an effort to strengthen their connection.

Although the suggested solutions offer a thorough method of addressing intimacy and expectations in romantic relationships, it's crucial to remember that every relationship is different and that some couples may benefit more from other approaches. Examining substitute approaches like consulting a professional counsellor, participating in couples counselling, or introducing personal self-care routines can provide other ways to deal with particular relationship problems.

Managing expectations and intimacy in love relationships is crucial to building a solid and long-lasting partnership. Consequently, the next segments will examine comprehensive tactics and useful resolutions for preserving closeness and skillfully handling anticipations in romantic partnerships, enabling partners to foster a satisfying and peaceful connection.

Traveling With Canker Sores

Traveling is a rewarding experience that enables people to discover new places, fully immerse themselves in other cultures, and make lifelong memories. However, the idea of travelling may pose particular difficulties for people who have canker sores. Aphthous ulcers, another name for canker sores, are excruciating oral ulcers that can cause discomfort when eating, drinking, and speaking. Taking preemptive steps and being well-prepared is necessary to manage canker sores during travel, making the experience seamless and pleasurable. People can reduce discomfort and make the most of their vacation experience by attending to the specific issues associated with canker sores.

The main concern when travelling with canker sores is the possibility of increased pain and discomfort, which can make the trip less enjoyable. It is possible for canker sores to be brought on by stress, exhaustion, and specific meals. Travel-related disturbances can also make it more likely that these ulcers would form or worsen. Canker sore discomfort can also make it difficult to enjoy regional cuisine, socialise with others, and fully partake in travel activities, which could negatively affect the entire trip experience.

The convenience and enjoyment of travelling may be greatly reduced if the difficulties associated with treating canker sores during travel are ignored. Increased discomfort from canker sores can make one less eager to explore, less willing to partake in gastronomic adventures, and less able to participate fully in social and cultural activities. Furthermore, the possibility of ongoing discomfort could cause annoyance and discontent, which would lower the level of enjoyment from the trip as a whole.

It is crucial to take preventative steps and bring necessities that can ease discomfort and make it easier to manage canker sores while travelling in order to lessen their effects. Travelers can reduce the disruptions caused by canker sores and maximise their enjoyment of the trip by implementing strategic solutions into their preparations.

Several crucial procedures must be taken in order to apply canker sore management strategies when travelling in order to reduce discomfort and facilitate efficient care. Before leaving on a trip, people should put together a thorough travel kit that includes specific dental care items, calming medications, and food suggestions that might lessen the effects of canker sores. Furthermore, while stress and fatigue are known to be triggers for canker sores, engaging in attentive self-care and making rest a priority while travelling can help lessen these conditions.

People can anticipate to feel less uncomfortable from canker sores if they diligently apply these remedies, which will allow them to enjoy their trip to the fullest. People can look forward to having more ability to enjoy regional foods, have meaningful conversations, and take part in trip activities without being limited by chronic mouth pain with cautious planning and proactive management. A more pleasurable and enriched travel experience as well as increased travel satisfaction are anticipated results of putting these solutions into practise.

Although the suggested remedies provide a thorough method for treating canker sores while travelling, it's crucial to recognise that every person's reaction and preference may differ. Additional options for efficiently managing canker sores and improving the travel experience include looking into alternate solutions like implementing stress-reduction techniques, consulting a healthcare provider for recommendations on specialised oral care, or changing eating habits while travelling.

Taking proactive measures to treat canker sores during travel is crucial to making the most out of the experience. As such, the ensuing parts will address thorough tactics and useful remedies for handling canker sores during travel, enabling people to reduce suffering and enjoy the experience to the fullest.

Canker Sores and Public Speaking

The ability to speak in front of an audience is crucial in both personal and professional settings. Effective and confident communication is highly regarded, whether one is giving speeches at special events or social gatherings or presenting presentations in the business sphere. Nevertheless, public speaking can pose serious difficulties for people who suffer from canker sores. Painful mouth ulcers known as canker sores can make it difficult to articulate words, make speaking uncomfortable, and lessen the impact and overall delivery of a speech or presentation. In order to preserve vocal health, reduce discomfort, and convey ideas with assurance and clarity, managing canker sores in the context of public speaking calls for particular tactics and concerns.

The main concern when speaking in public while suffering from canker sores is the possible damage to one's voice and the overall quality of the speech or presentation. Speaking with canker sores can be painful and uncomfortable, which can make it difficult to pronounce words clearly and consistently tone your voice. Furthermore, canker sores can cause self-consciousness and attention, which can hinder a speaker's ability to connect with the audience and effectively deliver their message. The speaker's goals, whether personal or professional, may be hampered as a result, and the speech's impact and effectiveness may be diminished.

The repercussions of not addressing the difficulties associated with managing canker sores during public speaking can have a major effect on the speaker's capacity to communicate with authority and confidence. Speaking while in pain due to canker sores can have a negative influence on the speech or presentation's overall efficacy as well as voice performance and audience engagement. Persistent discomfort and distraction can also contribute to emotions of uncertainty and self-doubt, which can make it harder for the speaker to convince the audience and leave a lasting impression.

The implementation of realistic solutions and procedures that help ease discomfort, maintain vocal health, and enhance successful communication is crucial in addressing the obstacles associated with speaking in public while suffering from canker sores. Through the use of focused remedies in the planning and performance of speeches or presentations, people can maximise their capacity to communicate effectively and talk with assurance even in the face of canker sores.

The management of canker sores during public speaking requires a multifaceted strategy that includes preventative measures as well as useful methods for preserving vocal health. People should prioritise good dental hygiene and use specialist oral care products that can reduce pain and accelerate the healing of canker sores before giving public speeches. In addition, even though canker sores can be uncomfortable, vocal exercises and mindfulness practises might support people in maintaining a steady and self-assured speaking voice. In order to reduce the effect of canker sores on their vocal performance, people can benefit from using strategic speaking strategies, such as tempo, emphasis, and modulation, during the speech or presentation.

People who faithfully apply these methods should be able to talk in public with less discomfort from canker sores, allowing them to communicate clearly and confidently. Even in the case of canker sores, people can still expect to be able to communicate more effectively and connect with the audience, make a compelling point, and leave a lasting impression. Despite the difficulties caused by canker sores, the expected results of putting these remedies into practise include better vocal performance, increased audience engagement, and the capacity to achieve goals connected to public speaking on a professional or personal level.

It's vital to recognise that while the suggested treatments provide a thorough strategy to managing canker sores during public speaking, individual responses and preferences may differ. Examining other options, such as consulting a speech therapist for advice on specific vocal care, using over-the-counter medications to relieve canker sore pain right away, or altering speech patterns to account for canker sores, can offer more options for successfully coping with the difficulties of giving public speeches while suffering from canker sores.

Proactively managing canker sores is crucial for maintaining vocal health and facilitating clear communication during public speaking. In order to enable people to speak confidently and effectively during public speaking even in the face of these mouth ulcers, the ensuing sections will explore thorough tactics and workable solutions for managing canker sores.

Pediatric Canker Sores: A Parent's Guide

Recognizing Canker Sores in Children

In order to properly diagnose and treat these oral lesions in children, parents and other caregivers must be familiar with the terminology related to canker sores. The goal of this chapter is to provide caregivers the knowledge they need to properly manage canker sore problems in children by providing a thorough guidance on how to identify them in children, distinguish them from other oral health issues, and more.

It's important to have a firm grasp of the terminology related to these oral lesions before diving into the detection of canker sores in children. To help with the identification and understanding of canker sores, the following concepts will be defined in this chapter: prodromal symptoms, oral mucosa, aphthous ulcers, canker sores, and differential diagnosis.

1. Canker Sores:

Phthous ulcers, another name for canker sores, are tiny, excruciating lesions that appear on the mucous membrane within the mouth. The tongue, gums, inner cheeks, and roof of the mouth can all develop these sores. Their round or oval form with a crimson border and a white or yellowish centre defines them. Canker sores are uncomfortable and irritating, especially when eating and talking. They can occur alone or in groups.

2. Aphthous Ulcers:

Phthalous ulcers are a prevalent form of oral lesion that are distinguished by their recurrent nature and correlation with variables including stress, hormone fluctuations, and specific diets. They are a worry for kids and their caregivers since they come in different sizes and frequently cause discomfort.

3. Oral Mucosa:

The term "oral mucosa" describes the mucous lining of the mouth, which includes the gums, cheeks, lips, and other soft tissues.

Recognizing irregularities like canker sores and telling them apart from other oral health disorders requires an understanding of the features of the oral mucosa.

4. Prodromal Symptoms:

Prodromal symptoms are the initial indications or feelings that come on before canker sores show up. A tingling or burning feeling at the location where the canker sore may eventually form is one of these signs. Caregivers can be informed of the potential presence of canker sores in children by identifying prodromal symptoms.

5. Differential Diagnosis:

Differential diagnosis is the process of identifying one illness from another by contrasting their unique traits and symptoms. When it comes to identifying canker sores in children, it is essential to comprehend the differential diagnostic process in order to correctly distinguish canker sores from other oral health conditions that may exhibit comparable symptoms.

To demonstrate how important it is to comprehend these phrases, picture a situation in which a child feels uncomfortable when they are eating. Understanding the jargon related to canker sores enables caregivers to explain symptoms appropriately, seek appropriate guidance for their child's oral health, and connect with healthcare specialists in an effective manner. Caregivers may confidently and clearly traverse the process of identifying canker sores in children by connecting these concepts to everyday situations.

Conclusion:

Recognizing and treating canker sores in children requires a basic understanding of the terminology associated with these oral lesions. Caregivers can equip themselves with the knowledge required to recognise canker sores and distinguish them from other oral health disorders by clearly defining essential concepts and their relevance. This will ultimately help with comprehensive management of canker sores in children.

Treatment Options for Children

Ensuring the well-being of children with canker sores requires a comprehensive understanding of safe and effective treatment options. This chapter covers a variety of therapeutic approaches, both conventional and non-traditional, that are especially created for patients in the paediatric population. Caregivers can effectively treat canker sores by carefully weighing all of the options, making educated judgments, and giving their kids proactive oral health care.

a. Children's canker sores frequently cause pain and suffering, thus topical analgesics should be applied to reduce symptoms and speed up the healing process. Benzocaine, lidocaine, or hydrogen peroxide-containing products can help by numbing the injured region and creating a healing environment. Children's canker sore outbreaks can be contained more quickly and with fewer side effects when antimicrobial medicines like chlorhexidine gluconate are used.

b. Adding mouthwashes and gentle oral rinses to a child's oral hygiene routine can help treat canker sores in addition to other methods. Mouthwashes with mild antiseptics, baking soda rinses, and saline solutions can help clear the oral cavity, lessen inflammation, and foster a healing environment. Choosing formulas free of alcohol is essential if you want to avoid needless irritation and pain.

b. The effect that dietary decisions have on the development of canker sores in children highlights the need of putting customised dietary changes into practise. Iron, folate, and vitamin B12-rich diets can help lessen the frequency and intensity of canker sore episodes. On the other hand, limiting acidic, spicy, and abrasive meals can help reduce inflammation and pain, creating an environment that is favourable for oral healing, and reducing the likelihood that young children will experience canker sore recurrence.

d. Since stress plays a role in the spread of canker sores, managing children with canker sores holistically requires including psychological support and stress-reduction strategies. Children coping with recurring canker sores can benefit from the application of techniques like mindfulness, relaxation techniques, and age-appropriate counselling, which can reduce stress-related triggers, increase emotional resilience, and provide a supportive atmosphere.

e. Adding specific nutritional supplements to a child's diet, such as zinc, L-lysine, and vitamin C, can strengthen the body's defences against infection and improve the health of the oral mucosa, which may lessen the frequency and intensity of bouts of canker sores. Additionally, adding probiotics—more especially, bifidobacterium and lactobacilli strains—can alter the oral microbiome, which may prevent the onset of canker sores and improve children's dental health in general.

f. Investigating complementary and alternative therapies for children's canker sores, such as acupuncture, herbal remedies, and homoeopathic preparations, can enhance traditional treatment methods. Even though there is conflicting data regarding the effectiveness of these therapies, some kids might benefit from the comprehensive approach and specialised care that alternative therapies offer, so their inclusion in an all-encompassing treatment plan that is adapted to each child's particular requirements is justified.

Clinical research has demonstrated the effectiveness of topical analgesics, such as lidocaine and benzocaine, in reducing pain in paediatric children who have canker sores. Furthermore, studies have shown how nutritional supplements, such as zinc and vitamin B12, may help reduce the frequency and intensity of childhood canker sore outbreaks. Testimonies from caregivers have demonstrated the palpable relief that children receive when stress management approaches and individualised food plans are implemented.

Adhering to age-appropriate dosages and applying topical analgesics and antibiotics with caution are necessary when incorporating them into a child's canker sore treatment plan. Teaching kids the value of using mouthwashes and rinses as part of their regular oral hygiene regimen encourages them to take an active role in maintaining their dental health. Working with a paediatric dietitian to create customised meal plans enables parents to maximise their child's nutritional consumption, which may reduce the frequency of canker sore breakouts. Providing age-appropriate activities and counselling sessions along with stress management strategies fosters children's emotional resilience and well-being while they face the obstacles presented by canker sores.

The multimodal approach to treating children's canker sores, which includes dietary changes, topical treatments, and psychological support, highlights how different modalities work together to promote holistic care. As we work through the nuances of each treatment option, it becomes clear that the best way to lessen the impact of canker sores on a kid's oral health and overall well-being is to take a comprehensive strategy that is customised to meet the specific needs of each child.

In conclusion, the variety of approaches to treating children's canker sores demonstrates the complex interactions between traditional and non-conventional modalities, all of which are motivated by the desire to improve children's dental health and general wellbeing. Caregivers can manage canker sores holistically and intelligently by adopting a nuanced awareness of various treatment choices and their useful uses. This will help them create an atmosphere that supports children's resilience and dental health at their best.

Communicating With Your Child's Healthcare Provider

Complete care for children with canker sores depends on effective communication between caregivers and healthcare professionals. Initiating a cooperative conversation with physicians and dentists equips caregivers with the information and direction they need to handle the intricacies of managing canker sores, encouraging proactive support for their kids' oral health and general wellbeing.

Healthcare practitioners may find it difficult to understand the subtleties of their child's illness and treatment preferences, which can make communicating canker sore concerns difficult. The absence of a systematic methodology in these conversations could hinder the achievement of customised treatment, hence jeopardising the effectiveness of canker sore treatment techniques for younger patients.

Insufficient communication between patients and healthcare professionals regarding issues related to canker sores may result in treatment outcomes that fall short of expectations, impeding prompt and focused management of children's canker sore episodes. Miscommunication can worsen the effects of canker sores on children's oral health and quality of life by underusing evidence-based therapies and ignoring unique factors impacting the development of canker sores.

Caregivers can use a systematic and knowledgeable approach to conversation, establishing a cooperative relationship with healthcare practitioners, in order to overcome the difficulties involved in sharing concerns about canker sores with paediatricians and dentists. Caregivers can actively participate in their child's care by using effective communication tactics. By doing so, they can offer insightful opinions and preferences that help create specialised plans for managing canker sores.

1. Caretakers can quickly summarise their child's history of canker sores, including the frequency, duration, and severity of episodes as well as any related symptoms, before scheduling medical appointments. Keeping track of how a child's canker sores affect their everyday activities and dental health can give medical professionals a thorough understanding of the condition.

2. Healthcare providers are urged to ask questions during consultations regarding evidence-based canker sore management alternatives. They should also clarify treatment techniques, possible side effects, and expected results. Promoting the use of holistic methods, like dietary adjustments and stress reduction strategies, can highlight the need of an all-encompassing treatment strategy.

3. Sharing decision-making with medical professionals allows parents to actively participate in their child's management strategy for canker sores. A collaborative partnership can be fostered by having conversations about treatment choices, follow-up evaluations, and long-term preventive plans. This will help to ensure that care is tailored to the child's specific requirements and family dynamics.

It has been demonstrated that structured and knowledgeable communication with healthcare providers improves the quality of care for young patients with chronic illnesses by making it easier to integrate patient preferences and execute evidence-based interventions in a customised way. Caregivers can help children with canker sores achieve better long-term outcomes in terms of treatment adherence, treatment satisfaction, and active participation in discourse and collaborative decision-making.

Seeking a second opinion from a paediatrician or consulting with a paediatric oral health specialist may provide additional perspectives and insights in situations where caregivers find it difficult to communicate concerns about canker sores with their child's primary healthcare provider. This reinforces the collaborative approach to managing canker sores.

Having good communication with medical professionals is crucial to maximising the treatment and wellbeing of kids with canker sores. Caregivers can advocate for comprehensive care that meets the diverse needs of children patients and confidently negotiate the difficulties of canker sore management by adopting structured and educated discussion.

Soothing Techniques for Children

It is crucial to teach children compassionate and efficient pain management measures while they are suffering from canker sores. The methods on this list are gentle ways that parents or other caregivers can use to help a child with canker sores feel better and heal more quickly. Through the application of these strategies, caregivers can offer children suffering from canker sores full support, thereby improving their oral health and general well-being.

Topical analgesic gels that numb the afflicted area, like those containing benzocaine or lidocaine, can relieve localised pain. These gels create a barrier of protection over the canker sore, lessening the child's suffering and irritation.

b. Dietary changes can have a major effect on a child's experience with canker sores. Reducing discomfort and accelerating recovery can be achieved by promoting the consumption of soft, non-irritating foods and steering clear of acidic or spicy foods. Moreover, maintaining sufficient consumption of vital nutrients, like iron and vitamin B12, supports general oral health.

c. Rinsing the mouth with a baking soda mixture or saline solution will help relieve discomfort, lessen inflammation, and clean out the canker sore. These solutions provide a calming impact on the affected region and are excellent for youngsters due to their soft nature.

d. Children can get over-the-counter pain relievers such as ibuprofen or acetaminophen as long as they follow the recommended dosage instructions. These drugs aid in the management of canker sore discomfort and may also lessen inflammation, enhancing comfort and making it easier for the youngster to eat and speak. The impact of stress on the development of canker sores and the severity of their symptoms can be reduced by implementing stress management techniques like mindfulness exercises, deep breathing exercises, or guided imagery. Caregivers can help create a supportive environment that promotes the child's general well-being by lowering their own stress levels.

Research has indicated that topical analgesic gels are effective in relieving pain associated with canker sores in younger people. Additionally, studies back up the use of dietary adjustments in the treatment of disorders affecting the oral mucosa, with a focus on the significance of nutrient intake for oral health and recovery. Furthermore, because of their calming and healing properties for canker sores, dental specialists have recommended the use of saline rinses and baking soda treatments.

The calming methods outlined above can be easily included by caregivers into the child's daily schedule to offer ongoing support. Caregivers can support a child's comfort and healing by making sure topical analgesic gels and painkillers are available, as well as by changing the child's diet to follow recommendations for dental health. Frequent application of stress-reduction methods encourages a comprehensive approach to the treatment of canker sores and enhances the child's general wellbeing.

It is critical for caregivers to understand how these methods are interconnected as they negotiate the application of various soothing techniques. The combination of several treatments is part of the holistic approach to managing canker sores, which guarantees total support for the child's oral health. A caring atmosphere that puts the comfort of the kid first and promotes healing can be created by caregivers by skillfully alternating between these tactics.

Nutritional Considerations for Kids

Examining the complex connection between dietary modifications and nutritional requirements is crucial for managing canker sores in kids. Nutrition has a complex effect on the onset and healing of canker sores, affecting aspects of immune response, tissue regeneration, and general oral health. Through an analysis of the unique nutritional requirements for kids suffering from canker sores, caregivers can get important knowledge about how to best use dietary approaches to mitigate symptoms and encourage recovery.

The management of canker sores in children and the promotion of oral health greatly depend on the dietary modifications and nutritional requirements customised for them.

The adequate intake of vital nutrients, especially vitamin B12 and iron, is one of the most important dietary factors for kids with canker sores. A lack of these micronutrients has been connected to a higher risk of oral mucosal disorders, such as canker sores, and is essential for preserving oral health. Iron aids in appropriate oxygen delivery and tissue repair within the oral cavity, while vitamin B12 is essential for immune system support and the regeneration of oral tissues.

Clinical research has demonstrated the importance of iron and vitamin B12 for maintaining dental health, as well as how they might lessen the frequency and severity of canker sores in young patients. Children who are deficient in these vital nutrients may experience longer healing times and repeated canker sores due to the compromised oral mucosa. In order to meet a child's nutritional needs and support their dental health, it is imperative that they include foods and supplements high in iron and vitamin B12.

Apart from the micronutrient aspects, it is important to pay attention to how dietary irritants and allergies affect the development of canker sores in children. Certain meals have been found to be possible causes for canker sores in sensitive individuals, including acidic fruits, spicy snacks, and chemicals that cause allergies. Caregivers can actively lessen the incidence and severity of canker sores in children, improving their comfort and well-being, by recognising and addressing certain dietary causes.

Although the management of canker sores is well-documented in relation to critical nutrients and dietary triggers, it is crucial to recognise the potential complexity of individual dietary responses. Different children might be more or less susceptible to the same food triggers, and the effects of nutritional treatments could differ depending on things like heredity, the quality of the child's diet overall, and any coexisting medical issues. Furthermore, a complete approach is required to effectively address canker sores in children due to the interplay between dietary modifications and other management measures, such as topical therapies and stress management.

Although individual responses may vary, there is still substantial data to support the impact of dietary triggers and important nutrients on the management of canker sores. Caregivers have a major role to play in reducing the incidence of canker sores and fostering dental health in children by placing a high priority on optimising the nutritional intake of their charges and proactively identifying and resolving dietary triggers. Furthermore, combining dietary concerns with other treatment methods enables a thorough and customised strategy that tackles the complex aspects of managing canker sores in young patients.

Probiotics may also have an impact on the development and severity of oral mucosal disorders, such as canker sores, by altering the oral microbiota and boosting oral immune function, according to recent studies. Adding probiotic-rich foods to a child's diet or taking supplements of probiotics is a promising way to improve dental health and reduce the symptoms of canker sores.

In summary, a key element of all-encompassing management approaches for kids with canker sores is their nutritional needs. Caregivers can actively help children with canker sores by addressing the sufficiency of vital nutrients, recognising and reducing dietary triggers, and investigating the possible advantages of probiotics. Their efforts can also help to reduce symptoms and improve oral health. The incorporation of these dietary factors into a comprehensive strategy for managing canker sores emphasises how important they are for enhancing the health of young patients.

Supporting Your Child's Emotional Health

A child's general health and quality of life are significantly impacted by their mental state when they have canker sores. Aphthous ulcers, another name for canker sores, can be extremely painful, distressing, and uncomfortable, especially in younger people. Beyond the physical symptoms, children with canker sores experience psychological effects that include emotional reactions including irritation, worry, and low self-esteem. Since canker sores have a direct impact on a child's mental and social development, it is imperative to recognise and address the emotional effects of the condition in order to provide comprehensive care for affected children.

The main concern here is the mental difficulties that kids have in dealing with canker sores. The mood, conduct, and social relationships of a kid may be affected by these oral lesions, which may result in increased emotional discomfort. Canker sore pain and discomfort can make a youngster irritable, reluctant to eat or speak, and possibly retreat from social situations. These behaviours might negatively impact the child's general emotional health.

A number of negative outcomes may result if the emotional impact of canker sores in children is not adequately treated. A youngster experiencing ongoing emotional discomfort may find it difficult to go about their everyday activities, do well in school, and establish and sustain healthy connections with peers and family members. Unmanaged emotional difficulties resulting from canker sores can also have long-term psychological implications, such as increased anxiety, decreased self-esteem, and a bad opinion of dental hygiene and self-care routines.

Children with canker sores require a multimodal strategy that incorporates psychological support, communication techniques, and coping skills in order to address their emotional well-being. It is feasible to lessen the detrimental emotional effects of canker sores and promote resilience and well-being in impacted children by giving them with appropriate emotional support and equipping caregivers with the required resources.

There are various essential elements that go into implementing emotional support techniques for kids who have canker sores. First and foremost, confirming the child's emotional experiences and offering comfort depend heavily on the caregivers, medical professionals, and the child having honest and compassionate communication. Using age-appropriate language and visual aids, educators may help children learn about canker sores and how to manage them. This can help reduce their anxiety and give them a sense of control over their condition. Furthermore, integrating relaxation methods, like deep breathing exercises or meditation, can help kids manage their discomfort and lessen the emotional anguish that comes with having canker sores.

There is evidence to support the idea that providing emotional support to kids who have canker sores improves their emotional health and coping skills. Children who receive all-encompassing emotional support exhibit increased resilience, decreased worry, and elevated self-esteem, which empowers them to face the difficulties presented by canker sores with increased flexibility and a more optimistic perspective. Effective emotional support also helps the kid continue with regular daily activities and social interactions, reducing the overall disturbance that canker sores create to the child's quality of life.

Although the suggested method places a strong emphasis on communication and psychological support, it is crucial to recognise the possible benefits of supplemental therapies as well. Other approaches, such paediatric cognitive-behavioral therapy, peer support groups, or art and play therapy, provide ways to approach the emotional effects of canker sores from other angles. By meeting the unique needs and preferences of impacted children, these non-traditional approaches to emotional support can supplement more established methods while also improving the overall efficacy of emotional care delivery.

In summary, children with canker sores require holistic care and management that places a high priority on their mental well. Caregivers and medical experts can help children manage their canker sores with resilience and positivity by identifying and treating the emotional difficulties they present. This will ultimately improve the children's emotional health and well-being.

Educating Peers and Caregivers

A crucial part of complete management of canker sores in children is educating peers and caregivers about the child's condition. Children with canker sores require a supportive, understanding, and accommodating environment, which is largely provided by peers and caregivers. To ensure that the kid receives the support and understanding they need, it is essential to promote effective communication and awareness among peers and caregivers. This will help to minimise the emotional and social effects that canker sores have on the child's well-being.

The main problem is that peers and caregivers do not know enough about the difficulties that children with canker sores encounter. This frequently results in misunderstandings, shame, and insufficient assistance, which has an impact on the child's social skills and emotional fortitude. Peers and caregivers may unintentionally exacerbate the child's mental discomfort if they are unaware of canker sores, which emphasises the importance of focused education and communication techniques.

Peers and caregivers may unintentionally cause insensitivity, social exclusion, and a lack of appropriate assistance if they continue to be unaware of or ignorant about a child's canker sore condition. Affected children may experience increased emotional distress, a reluctance to participate in social activities, and a sense of isolation as a result of this deficient comprehension. Additionally, because of what they perceive to be a lack of empathy and support from their immediate social circle, the youngster may suffer from heightened anxiety and low self-esteem.

Implementing an organised education and communication strategy with an emphasis on correct information, empathy, and useful ways to support the child with canker sores is the solution. This plan is directed towards peers and caregivers. Peers and caregivers can foster a more inclusive and supportive atmosphere that supports the child with canker sores by being equipped with the essential knowledge and communication skills.

A number of essential elements are required for the education and communication plan to be implemented. First and foremost, it's critical to educate children specifically about canker sores, dispelling myths and emphasising the condition's effects on the afflicted youngster. Informational meetings, the provision of educational resources, and participatory workshops with the goal of raising knowledge and comprehension can all help achieve this. Creating a supportive environment for a kid with canker sores also requires building sympathetic communication skills among classmates and caregivers. These abilities include active listening, validating the child's experiences, and offering emotional support.

Research suggests that good education and communication techniques for caregivers and peers have a positive impact on the emotional health and social integration of the kid. Youngsters who get support from a knowledgeable and compassionate social circle exhibit higher self-esteem, fewer feelings of loneliness, and a stronger sense of community among their peers. Additionally, a welcoming and encouraging atmosphere helps the child develop emotional resilience in general, which makes it easier for them to deal with their canker sore condition and has a favourable impact on their social relationships.

Although the suggested course of action focuses mostly on education and communication, it is important to take into account additional approaches to augment the care given to the child who has canker sores. Other options include the creation of caregiver support networks to enable the sharing of experiences, difficulties, and practical tips for caring for a child with canker sores, or peer education programmes where peers actively participate in learning about canker sores and supporting their affected classmates. By providing more opportunities for raising awareness and providing assistance within the kid's social ecology, these other options help create a more all-encompassing and long-lasting support network for the child.

In summary, it is critical to inform peers and caregivers about a child's canker sore condition in order to support the child's social integration and mental health. A loving environment that lessens the emotional burden of canker sores and promotes the child's holistic development and well-being can be established by encouraging understanding, empathy, and educated support within the child's social circle.

Advanced Topics in Canker Sore Research

Emerging Therapies

As we go deeper into the management of canker sores, it is critical to examine the novel therapies that have the potential to completely transform the way that this prevalent but problematic ailment is treated. Extensive study and testing have been conducted in an attempt to find effective treatments for canker sores, and the result has been the creation of novel strategies that may be able to address the underlying causes and reduce symptoms. We will examine the effectiveness of new treatments for canker sores and how they might affect the treatment of this ailment in this chapter.

There is some promise for more thorough and successful care of canker sores with the introduction of novel and experimental therapies.

Probiotic usage is one of the most promising new treatments for canker sores. Studies have shown that some probiotic strains, especially Lactobacillus reuteri, have the ability to alter the oral microbiota and lower the risk of canker sores. Research has shown that giving L. reuteri to people who are prone to recurring episodes significantly reduced both the frequency and severity of canker sores. The aforementioned primary evidence highlights the possibility of probiotics as a feasible therapeutic strategy for the management of canker sores.

The microbial equilibrium that is restored in the oral cavity by probiotics is the mechanism by which they are effective in reducing the incidence of canker sores. Probiotics provide a focused way to treat the oral microbiome imbalances that have been connected to the onset and aggravation of canker sores. Probiotics produce an environment less conducive to the production of canker sores by encouraging the growth of good bacteria and inhibiting the proliferation of harmful microorganisms. Additionally, some probiotic strains have anti-inflammatory qualities that help to lessen inflammation of the oral mucosa, which helps to lessen the symptoms of canker sores. This comprehensive review confirms that probiotics have the potential to be an effective new treatment for canker sores.

Some research has shown contradictory results, despite the encouraging discoveries about the effectiveness of probiotics in the treatment of canker sores. There have been concerns raised over the consistency of the therapeutic effects due to several trials reporting little to no improvement in the prevalence of canker sores after probiotic intervention. Furthermore, individual differences in the composition of their oral microbiomes and the impact of several variables including nutrition and dental hygiene habits could lead to variations in how well a person responds to probiotic therapy. These counterarguments highlight how difficult it is to treat canker sores universally using probiotics.

Even while there is room for variation in the response to probiotics, it is important to recognise the complexity of each person's microbial profile and the requirement for tailored methods when putting probiotic therapy into practise. In addition, current investigations are concentrated on clarifying the elements that lead to the varied reaction to probiotics in order to improve the standards for choosing the best candidates. Probiotics have the potential to be an effective developing therapy for canker sores; however, this can only be fully realised by resolving the constraints and improving the therapeutic procedures.

Apart from probiotics, recent studies have also brought attention to the possibility of photobiomodulation therapy for the treatment of canker sores. Photobiomodulation, which makes use of particular light wavelengths, has shown anti-inflammatory and wound-healing properties. This means that it provides a tailored, non-invasive method of treating canker sores. Initial investigations have demonstrated encouraging outcomes, indicating the need for additional investigation into this novel treatment as an adjunctive approach to the treatment of canker sores.

In summary, research into new treatments for canker sores reveals a landscape teeming with viable answers that could completely alter the way that these lesions are treated. The data demonstrating the effectiveness of probiotics and the potential of photobiomodulation therapy, despite obstacles and unknowns, highlight how revolutionary these new treatments are for the treatment of canker sores. The possibility of attaining thorough and efficient care of canker sores is becoming more real as research advances and creative strategies are honed, providing hope to those who struggle with this recurrent ailment.

Genetic Studies and Personalized Medicine

The endeavour to grasp the intricacies involved in managing canker sores has prompted a comprehensive investigation into genetic studies and their possible consequences for customised treatment approaches. The field of genetic research is showing us that the use of genetic knowledge to customised treatment has the potential to completely transform the way that canker sores are managed. In the context of managing canker sores, this chapter provides a thorough examination of the interactions between genetic research and personalised medicine, illuminating prospective paths for specialised interventions and precision treatments.

By incorporating genetic research into personalised medicine, it may be possible to develop tailored therapy regimens for the management of canker sores, leading to a new level of accuracy and effectiveness in the treatment of this recurrent illness.

The complex interactions between genetic predispositions and the clinical presentation of canker sores provide the basis for utilising genetic studies in personalised medicine for the treatment of this ailment. Strong evidence has been found through research connecting certain genetic differences to a higher risk of developing recurring canker sores. The development and severity of canker sores are influenced by genetic loci linked to immunological modulation, inflammation, and oral mucosal integrity, as revealed by genome-wide association studies. The foundation for incorporating genetic insights into customised therapy plans for the management of canker sores is laid by these main findings.

Canker sores have complex genetic roots, which highlights the possibility for personalised medicine to customise treatments according to individual genetic profiles. Personalized medicine can help identify tailored therapy methods that target the precise molecular pathways implicated in the pathophysiology of canker sores by clarifying the genetic elements that contribute to an individual's susceptibility to the ailment. Additionally, by incorporating genetic information into the decision-making process for therapy, interventions like immunomodulatory therapies, targeted pharmaceuticals, and dietary changes can be tailored to each patient's specific genetic responses and susceptibilities. This comprehensive analysis highlights the revolutionary potential of genetic insights in creating individualised therapy regimens for the management of canker sores.

Despite the potential benefits of using genetic research for personalised medicine in the treatment of canker sores, it is important to recognise the difficulties and complications involved in converting genetic discoveries into practical treatment plans. Rebuttals emphasise how canker sore formation is multifaceted, involving genetic predispositions interacting with oral microbiota, lifestyle choices, and environmental factors. The complex interactions among these several components could make it difficult to pinpoint the exact roles that genetic factors play in canker sore susceptibility and severity. This would cast doubt on the viability of using genetic data alone to inform individualised therapies.

Although canker sores are complicated and require careful consideration of lifestyle and environmental factors, genetic findings are rarely used in isolation in personalised treatment. Instead, it provides a sophisticated understanding of the genetic foundations that might guide focused interventions, enhancing current knowledge and diagnostic techniques. Additionally, developments in computational analyses and bioinformatics make it possible to combine genetic, environmental, and clinical data to create comprehensive risk profiles. This makes it easier to identify individualised treatment plans that take into account the intricate interactions between environmental factors and genetic predispositions.

Apart from the clarification of genetic predispositions, recent studies have revealed the possibility of utilising pharmacogenomic insights to customise pharmaceutical therapies for the management of canker sores. Individual responses to pharmacological drugs routinely employed in the management of canker sores can be influenced by genetic variations in immune response genes and drug metabolic pathways. Personalized medicine can improve drug selection, dosing schedules, and therapeutic outcomes by utilising pharmacogenomic data. This can maximise the effectiveness of pharmacological therapies while reducing the risk of side effects.

In summary, the promise of customised therapies that are in line with each patient's unique genetic susceptibilities and reactions signals a paradigm shift in the management of canker sores brought about by the incorporation of genetic studies into personalised medicine. Precision therapies that address the multifaceted character of canker sores may be informed by the synthesis of genetic, environmental, and clinical data, notwithstanding the difficulties and complexities involved in converting genetic insights into practicable treatment regimens. The possibility of customised treatment plans for the management of canker sores is becoming more real as research endeavours continue to elucidate the complex genetic foundations and improve the applications of personalised medicine. This will open the door to a new era of accuracy and effectiveness in treating this recurrent condition.

The Microbiome and Canker Sores

Gaining insight into the complex interplay between the oral microbiota and the onset of canker sores could be extremely beneficial in illuminating the underlying processes that contribute to the pathophysiology of this recurrent illness. An intricate ecology made up of many microbial communities, the oral microbiome is essential for preserving oral health and regulating immunological responses in the oral cavity. In order to better understand the potential implications for customised interventions and precision medicines based on the microbial composition and dynamics within the oral environment, this chapter will explore the relationship between the oral microbiome and canker sores.

The development and severity of canker sores are closely associated with the makeup and dynamics of the oral microbiome. This suggests a promising avenue for tailored therapies and focused treatment strategies that capitalise on the knowledge gained from the oral microbial environment.

A growing corpus of studies has clarified how the oral microbiota affects a person's susceptibility to the appearance of canker sores. Research has demonstrated changes in the diversity and makeup of microorganisms in the oral environments of people who experience recurrent canker sores, pointing to a possible link between the development of dysbiotic microbial communities and the start of this illness. Research on the oral microbiome has also revealed the existence of particular microbial taxa and their interactions, which may be involved in the development and maintenance of oral mucosal inflammation, a characteristic that is characteristic of canker sores. These key findings establish the groundwork for incorporating microbial insights into customised treatment approaches and highlight the role of the oral microbiome in determining the pathophysiological landscape of canker sores.

The complex relationship between canker sores and the oral microbiome goes beyond the taxonomic makeup of microbial communities to include the functional characteristics and metabolic processes of the oral microbiota. Canker sore aetiology has been linked to dysbiotic changes in microbial functions, including dysregulation of oral mucosal immune responses and disruptions in immune-modulatory metabolite synthesis. The oral microbiome's dynamic interaction with host immune cells, such as epithelial cells and resident immunological populations, highlights the potential impact on the onset and severity of canker sores. Personalized therapies can be designed to modify microbial functions and restore a balanced oral ecosystem by exploring the functional characteristics of the oral microbiome. This will help to mitigate the risk of recurrent canker sores.

Despite strong evidence linking the oral microbiome to the pathophysiology of canker sores, it is important to recognise the intricate nature of the oral microbial ecosystem and the variety of factors that could obscure the causal relationships between individual microbial taxa and the development of canker sores. The oral cavity's microbial dysbiosis is multifactorial, according to counterarguments. The oral microbiome is shaped by a combination of systemic health issues, dietary habits, environmental factors, and oral hygiene practises. This intricacy calls into doubt the specificity and causation of microbial imbalances in causing canker sores to develop and reoccur. As a result, a thorough analysis of the wider contextual factors influencing oral microbial dynamics is necessary.

The integration of microbial insights into tailored interventions acknowledges the multivariate character of the oral microbiome and avoids oversimplifying the intricate dynamics of the oral microbial ecology. Instead, it provides a more nuanced understanding of the functional characteristics and microbial interactions that may affect a person's susceptibility to canker sores. This understanding allows for the development of targeted strategies that alter the oral microbiome in order to improve oral health and reduce the likelihood of recurrent canker sores. Moreover, developments in computational analyses and high-throughput sequencing technologies enable the thorough characterization of the oral microbiome, including its taxonomic, functional, and ecological aspects. This comprehensive perspective takes into account the complex interactions between microbial, environmental, and host factors in the context of managing canker sores.

Emerging research has revealed the possibility of probiotic interventions and microbiome-targeted therapeutics in restoring oral microbial balance and lessening the severity of canker sores, in addition to the dysbiotic modifications in the oral microbiome. Probiotic formulations with beneficial microbial strains have demonstrated potential in improving oral mucosal integrity and altering the oral microbial habitat, which in turn lowers the frequency and length of canker sore episodes. Furthermore, novel approaches to reestablishing a eubiotic oral microbiome and mitigating the disruptions linked to recurring canker sores are provided by the understanding gained from microbiome-targeted medicines, such as microbial transplantation and microbial metabolite supplementation.

In summary, the relationship between the oral microbiome and canker sores is a critical pathway for tailored interventions and targeted treatments that leverage the knowledge gained from the oral microbial ecology. While acknowledging the intricate and multifaceted nature of the oral microbiome, tailored strategies that address the dysbiotic alterations and functional characteristics of the oral microbiome in the context of managing canker sores may be informed by the synthesis of microbial insights with clinical and environmental data. The prospect of using microbial insights for personalised treatment plans is becoming more real as research endeavours continue to untangle the complex microbial underpinnings and refine the applications of personalised medicine. This will open the door to a new era of accuracy and effectiveness in managing the recurrent nature of canker sores.

Immunotherapy and Canker Sores

The investigation of immunotherapy in the management of canker sores marks a potentially fruitful avenue for the discovery of new treatment approaches and prophylactic measures. Immunotherapy presents a promising approach to addressing the underlying immunological dysregulation linked to the pathophysiology of canker sores. It is defined by the targeted control of immune responses to elicit specific therapeutic effects. This chapter attempts to explore the possibilities of immunotherapy for the treatment of canker sores, illuminating the immunological complexities and therapeutic implications that support this novel strategy.

Immunotherapy presents a personalised and effective treatment option that goes beyond traditional symptomatic management of canker sores by potentially modifying aberrant immune responses and reducing the recurrent nature of this condition.

A growing corpus of studies has shown the critical role that immunological dysregulation plays in the development and progression of canker sores. According to immunological studies, the oral mucosa exhibits aberrant immune responses that are typified by dysregulated cytokine profiles, altered immune cell dynamics, and disruptions in immune regulatory pathways. The aforementioned discoveries not only illustrate the immunopathological terrain of canker sores but also underscore the complex interaction between innate and adaptive immune elements in moulding the pathophysiological environment beneath this recurrent ailment. Furthermore, the discovery of distinct immunological markers linked to canker sores offers a strong basis for utilising immunotherapeutic approaches to restore immune equilibrium and lessen the vulnerability to recurring ulcerative lesions in the oral cavity.

The pathophysiological mechanisms of canker sores are not limited to immune response dysregulation; they also involve the interaction of immune cells, inflammatory mediators, and the oral mucosal milieu. The inflammatory cascades that are typical of canker sores have been linked to dysbiotic changes in immune cell populations, specifically T lymphocytes, and their effector roles. The recurrent nature of canker sores is further highlighted by the dysregulated expression of pro-inflammatory cytokines, such as tumour necrosis factor-alpha (TNF-α) and interleukin-1β (IL-1β), as well as the disrupted activity of immune regulatory pathways, such as regulatory T cell-mediated immunomodulation. Through an exploration of the immunopathological aspects, immunotherapy becomes apparent as a focused method to regulate immune dysregulation and reestablish immune homeostasis, consequently tackling the fundamental immunological disruptions linked to canker sores.

In light of the strong data defining the immunopathogenesis of canker sores, it is critical to recognise the intricacy of immune dysregulation in the oral mucosa as well as the variety of variables that contribute to the complicated immunological environment. Rebuttals highlight the multifaceted character of immunological dysregulation, in which a combination of genetic susceptibility, environmental stressors, and systemic immune disruptions shapes the immunopathological environment linked to canker sores. Furthermore, the efficacy and specificity of immunotherapeutic interventions in modifying the various aspects of immune dysregulation demand careful thought, especially when it comes to customised immunotherapeutic strategies based on unique immunological profiles.

The incorporation of immunotherapy into the care of canker sores acknowledges the multifaceted nature of immunological dysregulation in canker sores and provides a focused and sophisticated approach to rebalance immune homeostasis, without oversimplifying the complexity of immunopathogenesis. Immunotherapy, which includes a variety of therapies from immuno-modulatory drugs to targeted biologics, has the capacity to target the various aspects of immune dysregulation associated with canker sores, providing customised approaches that go beyond standard symptomatic care. Additionally, developments in personalised medicine and immunological profiling enable the identification of certain immunotherapeutic modalities that correspond with individual immunological signatures, opening the door for precision immunotherapy in the context of managing canker sores.

Apart from defining immunopathological mechanisms, recent studies have shown how immune-modulatory drugs, like corticosteroids and immunomodulators, can reduce the severity and recurrence of canker sores by focusing on particular immune pathways. Additionally, the development of biologic therapies—such as monoclonal antibodies that target immune cell populations and pro-inflammatory cytokines—offers a customised and effective immunotherapeutic strategy that may be able to correct immune dysregulation and lessen the risk of recurrent canker sores. These novel approaches highlight the potential of immunotherapy in the management of canker sores and open the door to precision immunotherapeutic therapies tailored to the unique immunopathological profiles of patients suffering from this ailment.

Finally, the application of immunotherapy to the treatment of canker sores provides a novel approach to targeting the underlying immunopathological dysregulation and reducing the recurrent character of this illness. By carefully adjusting immune responses and readjusting immunological homeostasis, immunotherapy provides a customised and effective method that goes beyond traditional symptomatic treatment, ushering in a new era of accuracy and effectiveness in the treatment of canker sores. The prospect of using immune insights for customised treatment plans is becoming more real as research endeavours to better understand the immunological mechanisms underlying canker sores and improve the applications of personalised immunotherapy. This will likely lead to a paradigm shift in the management of canker sores.

Regenerative Medicine and Healing

The use of regenerative medicine to the treatment of canker sores is a significant opportunity to clarify novel therapeutic approaches intended to promote immune regulation, tissue regeneration, and repair of the oral mucosa. Regenerative medicine presents a compelling paradigm for addressing the tissue-level perturbations and immunological dysregulation linked to the pathogenesis and persistence of canker sores. It is distinguished by its emphasis on utilising both exogenous regenerative modalities and endogenous reparative mechanisms. The goal of this chapter is to examine the possibilities of regenerative medicine in the context of managing canker sores, illuminating the therapeutic implications and complexities of regenerative medicine that support this forward-thinking strategy.

Regenerative medicine has great potential to promote tissue healing, regulate abnormal immune responses, and lessen the recurrent nature of canker sores. As a result, it presents a comprehensive and regenerative treatment option that goes beyond traditional symptomatic care.

A growing corpus of studies has shown the critical role that tissue disruptions and compromised healing processes play in the development and maintenance of canker sores. Histological analyses have demonstrated aberrant tissue architecture, impaired epithelial integrity, and dysregulated wound healing dynamics in the oral mucosa. These findings underscore the complex interaction between immune dysregulation and tissue-level perturbations in determining the pathophysiological environment responsible for this recurrent ailment. Furthermore, the discovery of certain regenerative approaches and healing pathways linked to canker sores offers a strong basis for utilising regenerative medicine to promote tissue healing, reestablish mucosal balance, and lessen the likelihood of recurring ulcerative lesions in the oral cavity.

The regeneration details involved in the pathophysiology of canker sores go beyond simple tissue-level disruptions and include the interactions of immune regulation, reparative signalling pathways, and the oral mucosal milieu. Canker sores are recurrent due to a variety of complex regenerative aberrations, including dysregulated expression of growth factors like epidermal growth factor (EGF) and transforming growth factor-beta (TGF-β) and disrupted activity of reparative pathways like extracellular matrix remodelling and epithelial restitution. Through exploring the regenerative dimensions, regenerative medicine becomes apparent as a comprehensive strategy to support mucosal healing, modulate immune dysregulation, and facilitate tissue repair—all of which help address the immunological dysregulation and underlying tissue-level perturbations that are linked to canker sores.

Considering the strong data that outlines the regeneration details of canker sores, it is critical to recognise the intricacy of tissue disruptions in the oral mucosa as well as the variety of elements that contribute to the complicated regenerative and immunological environment. While genetic predisposition, local microenvironmental cues, and systemic regulatory systems all have a role in establishing the regenerative and immunological milieu associated with canker sores, counterarguments highlight the multifaceted nature of poor healing processes. Furthermore, the specificity and effectiveness of regenerative interventions in modifying the various aspects of tissue disruptions and immunological dysregulation demand careful thought, especially when it comes to customised regenerative strategies catered to unique immunological and regenerative profiles.

The integration of regenerative medicine into canker sore management acknowledges the multifactorial nature of tissue perturbations and immune dysregulation in canker sores, but does not oversimplify the complexities of regenerative and immunopathogenesis. Rather, it offers a comprehensive and nuanced approach to promote mucosal healing, modulate immune homeostasis, and foster tissue repair. Regenerative medicine, which includes a variety of interventions from tissue engineering techniques to reparative biologics, has the capacity to tackle the various aspects of tissue disruptions and immunological dysregulation associated with canker sores, providing all-encompassing approaches that go beyond traditional symptomatic treatment. Precision regenerative medicine in the context of managing canker sores is made possible by developments in regenerative profiling and customised medicine, which enable the identification of certain restorative modalities that correspond with unique regenerative and immunological signatures.

Apart from defining tissue-level disruptions, recent studies have shown how regenerative approaches, like growth factor-based treatments and tissue-engineered constructs, can promote tissue healing, restore mucosal balance, and lessen the severity and recurrence of canker sores by focusing on particular immune and regenerative pathways. Moreover, the development of regenerative biologics—such as mesenchymal stem cell therapies and platelet-rich plasma—offers a complete and regenerative strategy that may be useful in promoting mucosal repair, recalibrating tissue disturbances, and modifying immunological dysregulation. These cutting-edge techniques not only highlight the potential of regenerative medicine in the treatment of canker sores, but they also open the door to precision regenerative interventions that are tailored to the unique immunopathological and regenerative characteristics of those who suffer from this condition.

In summary, regenerative medicine's incorporation into canker sore treatment offers a revolutionary approach to addressing the underlying tissue-level disruptions, promoting mucosal repair, and reducing the recurrent nature of this illness. Regenerative medicine heralds a new era of precision and efficacy in the management of canker sores by providing a customised and effective approach that goes beyond traditional symptomatic management. This is achieved through comprehensive strategies that include tissue repair, immune modulation, and regenerative therapeutics. The field of canker sore management is about to undergo a paradigm shift as research endeavours to better understand the regenerative underpinnings of canker sores and refine the applications of personalised regenerative medicine continue to yield tangible results. One such application is the possibility of utilising regenerative insights for customised treatment plans.

International Approaches to Canker Sores

Phthous ulcers, another name for canker sores, are a common oral mucosal ailment that can occur on the inside of the lips, cheeks, or other parts of the oral cavity. These lesions are painful and superficial. The disorder has a substantial negative influence on oral health and quality of life. Its symptoms include increased sensitivity to foods that are acidic, spicy, or abrasive, as well as discomfort when eating and speaking. Canker sores are recurrent, which emphasises the need for efficient management techniques to reduce symptoms, encourage healing, and lessen the frequency of ulcerative episodes.

It is crucial to take into account the various cultural, socioeconomic, and healthcare contexts that impact how this ailment is seen, treated, and how results are achieved when examining global approaches to managing canker sores. Comprehensive and culturally sensitive methods to canker sore management can be informed by contrasting and comparing canker sore management practises across various cultures and healthcare systems.

In order to identify culturally sensitive tactics, treatment modalities, and healthcare paradigms that could improve the all-encompassing management of canker sores, this comparative analysis aims to clarify the subtleties and wider implications of canker sore management across international contexts. This investigation aims to provide insights on the various regimens, cultural beliefs, and healthcare systems that influence the experiences and outcomes of people coping with canker sores worldwide by comparing and contrasting approaches to the condition's management.

The benchmarks for comparison will cover the medical, cultural, and societal aspects of managing canker sores, including but not restricted to medical interventions, traditional remedies, accessibility to healthcare, and the application of regenerative medicine or other cutting-edge therapeutic modalities. To give a comprehensive evaluation of the global responses to this problem, the impact of cultural beliefs, stigmatisation, and the infrastructure of oral healthcare on the management of canker sores will also be taken into account.

Analyzing the commonalities between global methods to the treatment of canker sores reveals that traditional medicines are frequently important in a variety of cultural situations. To reduce symptoms and encourage the healing of canker sores, herbal remedies, topical applications of natural agents, and conventional treatment techniques are commonly used. These methods demonstrate a common focus on natural and culturally entrenched therapeutic approaches.

Furthermore, the incorporation of novel therapeutic approaches and regenerative medicine is becoming more popular in different healthcare systems across borders, providing promising paths for all-encompassing management of canker sores. The understanding of the immunological dysregulation and regenerative complexities that underlie canker sores has prompted research into regenerative modalities as a way to promote tissue repair, regulate aberrant immune responses, and lessen the recurrent nature of this condition. This represents a convergence in the search for cutting-edge therapeutic paradigms.

Even though regenerative medicine has been integrated with traditional medicines, there are still significant discrepancies in the affordability and accessibility of managing canker sores in various cultural and healthcare contexts. Reliance on traditional treatments in resource-constrained environments may be influenced by financial hardships and restricted access to official healthcare, which in turn shapes the prevalent treatment modalities and healthcare-seeking behaviours. This is in contrast to areas with developed healthcare systems, where people could have easier access to specialised dental care, medical interventions, and regenerative therapies for the treatment of canker sores.

Moreover, the disclosure of canker sores and the use of official healthcare services can be influenced by cultural attitudes and the shame associated with oral disorders. Certain cultures may have taboos or beliefs around canker sores, which makes people turn to traditional or alternative therapies instead of seeking professional medical attention. This cultural variance in beliefs and methods of seeking medical attention highlights the various sociocultural factors that affect canker sore management in various global contexts.

The reader's comprehension of the subtle differences and similarities in global approaches to canker sore management can be improved by using visual aids such as illustrations of traditional remedies, regenerative interventions, and healthcare infrastructure to highlight the comparative features of canker sore management in various cultural and healthcare contexts.

A comparative study of different countries' efforts to managing canker sores reveals the complex interactions between healthcare, social, and cultural elements that influence how people with this ailment experience and recover. In order to address the complex aspects of canker sore management, it emphasises the value of culturally sensitive and all-encompassing approaches that take into account conventional treatments, regenerative interventions, and healthcare accessibility. Moreover, the insights gathered from this comparison underline the necessity for culturally sensitive and fair treatments that suit the different beliefs, healthcare infrastructures, and socioeconomic realities that influence canker sore management on a worldwide scale.

Given the increased awareness of the global burden of oral diseases and the need to promote oral health equity, this comparative analysis is still relevant today. Healthcare professionals, legislators, and public health advocates can customise interventions, healthcare policies, and educational programmes to address the various needs and difficulties related to canker sore management across various cultural and healthcare contexts by having a thorough understanding of the global approaches to canker sore management. Moreover, the knowledge gathered from this analysis can guide joint initiatives to enhance the affordability, accessibility, and cultural suitability of canker sore care, supporting all-encompassing and inclusive approaches to oral health globally.

Conclusively, the comparative examination of global strategies for managing canker sores sheds light on the complex aspects of this ailment in various cultural and medical contexts. Through a comprehensive analysis of the parallels and divergences in conventional treatments, stem cell therapies, healthcare accessibility, and sociocultural factors, this investigation provides significant understanding of the subtleties and wider consequences of managing canker sores worldwide. It emphasises how crucial it is to develop inclusive oral healthcare solutions that cut across geographic and cultural divides by taking a holistic, egalitarian, and culturally sensitive approach to meeting the various needs and realities of those impacted by canker sores.

Future Directions in Canker Sore Management

A great deal of clinical investigation and study has been conducted on the treatment of canker sores, also referred to as aphthous ulcers. It is important to make predictions about how canker sore treatment may change in the future and what that will mean for individuals who suffer from this recurrent oral mucosal ailment as the medical and dentistry sciences advance. This chapter attempts to explore possible future paths in the treatment of canker sores, taking into account new therapeutic modalities, technological advancements, and interdisciplinary approaches that could change the way people with canker sores are cared for.

Personalized and precision-based therapies that address the underlying immunological dysregulation, promote tissue repair, and lessen the recurrent nature of aphthous ulcers are promising for the therapy of canker sores in the future. Additionally, the management of canker sores is about to undergo a revolution thanks to the integration of digital health technologies, regenerative medicine, and comprehensive oral healthcare paradigms. These approaches will provide patients with a variety of options for symptom relief, healing promotion, and improved quality of life.

Precision medicine methods may be used to treat canker sores as emerging therapy modalities such targeted biologics and immunomodulatory drugs show promise in preclinical and clinical investigations. Through targeted mechanisms, these therapies seek to moderate aberrant immune responses, reduce mucosal inflammation, and facilitate the healing of canker sores. This represents a paradigm change toward individualised treatment plans based on each patient's unique immunological profile.

The development of precision medicine in the treatment of canker sores involves the discovery of certain molecular targets and immune pathways involved in the aetiology of aphthous ulcers. Through deciphering the immunogenetic foundations of canker sores, scientists are identifying new treatment avenues that interact with the complex immunological pathways responsible for mucosal inflammation and ulcer formation. The development of biologics and small compounds that specifically target the dysregulated immunological milieu and provide customised therapies to address the varied character of canker sores is made possible by this profound understanding of the immunopathogenesis of the disorder.

Precision medicine is full of promise, but there are obstacles in the way of its widespread application in the therapy of canker sores. These include the high cost of targeted biologics, the need for significant clinical validation, and regulatory approvals. Furthermore, in order to stratify patients and optimise the selection of targeted therapies, the multifactorial aetiology of canker sores and the complexities of individual immune responses demand comprehensive profiling approaches, which may present logistical and resource-related challenges in clinical practise.

The identification of biomarkers, immunophenotypes, and genetic signatures linked to canker sore susceptibility and severity is being made easier by continuous developments in high-throughput omics technologies, bioinformatics, and computational modelling, despite the difficulties that precision medicine entails. These discoveries not only provide pathways for the classification of patients and the prediction of treatment outcomes, but they also propel the creation of economical profiling techniques that can be incorporated into standard clinical procedures to direct the prudent application of immunomodulatory drugs and targeted biologics in the treatment of canker sores.

Regenerative modalities, such as tissue engineering, stem cell therapies, and growth factor applications, are becoming more and more popular as possible supplements to traditional methods in the treatment of canker sores, in addition to precision medicine. Preclinical research has shown that these treatments have the capacity to regenerate by facilitating mucosal healing, reducing ulcerative symptoms, and altering the immunomodulatory environment in the oral mucosa. This suggests an additional treatment option for the overall treatment of canker sores.

Finally, the management of canker sores in the future has enormous promise for tailored, regenerative, and precision-based approaches that target the various immunopathogenic pathways and clinical presentations of aphthous ulcers. Even though there are obstacles in the way of putting these novel ideas into practise, the changing field of medicine and dentistry provides a compelling path for redefining the treatment of patients with canker sores by promoting individualised, regenerative, and comprehensive approaches that go beyond the status quo. Patients suffering from canker sores stand to gain from multimodal, patient-centered treatments that relieve their symptoms, advance dental health, and improve their general well-being when these future directions become practical reality.

Printed in the USA
CPSIA information can be obtained
at www.ICGtesting.com
LVHW010521121124
796309LV00001BA/152